shiatsu

D0516825

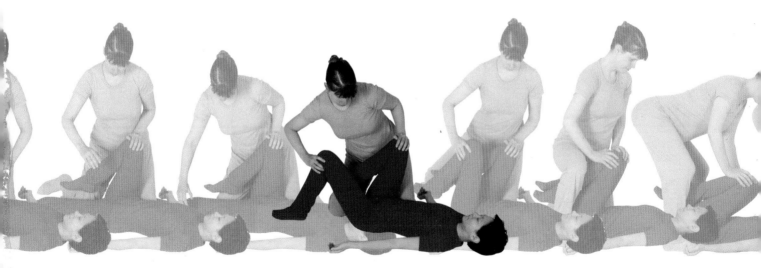

a *flow**motion*™ title

shiatsu

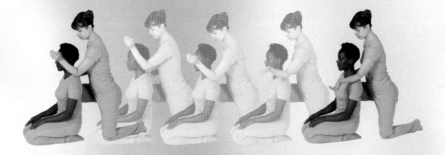

daisy cole

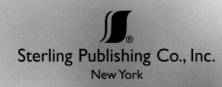

Sterling Publishing Co., Inc.
New York

Created and conceived by
Axis Publishing Limited
8c Accommodation Road
London NW11 8ED
www.axispublishing.co.uk

Creative Director: Siân Keogh
Managing Editor: Brian Burns
Design: Axis Design Editions
Project Editor: Conor Kilgallon
Production Manager: Sue Bayliss
Production Controller: Juliet Brown

Photographer: Mike Good

Library of Congress Cataloging-in-Publication Data
Available

10 9 8 7 6 5 4 3 2 1

Published in 2003 by Sterling Publishing Co., Inc.
387 Park Avenue South, New York, NY 10016
Text and images © Axis Publishing Limited 2003
Distributed in Canada by Sterling Publishing
c/o Canadian Manda Group,
One Atlantic Avenue, Suite 105
Toronto, Ontario, Canada, M6K 3E7

Every effort has been made to ensure that all the
information in this book is accurate. However, due to
differing conditions, and individual skills, the publisher
cannot be responsible for any injuries, losses, and other
damages which may result from the use of the
information in this book.

All rights reserved. No part of this book may be
reproduced in any form, by photostat, microfilm,
xerography, or any other means, or incorporated into any
retrieval system, electronic or mechanical, without the
written permission of the copyright owner.

Printed by Star Standard (Pte) Limited

ISBN 0–8069–9378–2

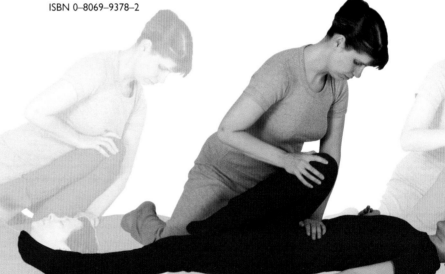

a *flowmotion*™ title

shiatsu

contents

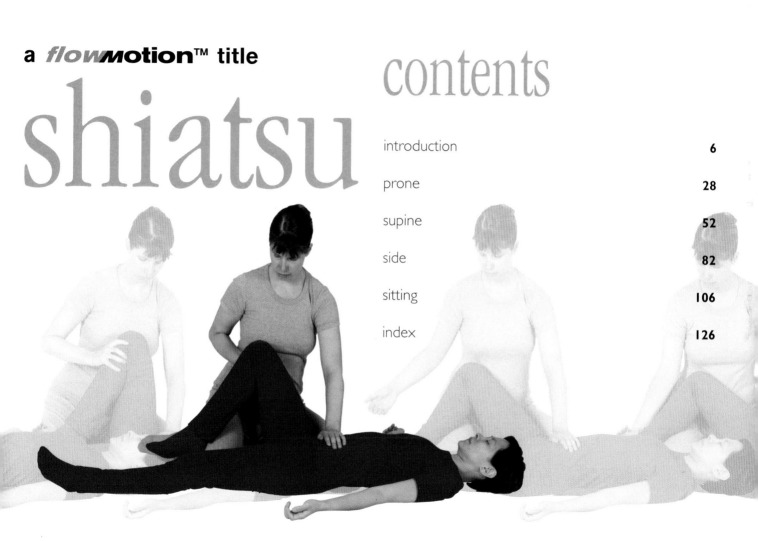

what is shiatsu?

Shiatsu is an ancient healing art from Japan that literally translates as "finger pressure." More importantly, it provides us with a way of getting to know our true selves through the sensation of touch. This touch should be safe and supportive, like the hands of a good friend in times of need, making us feel nurtured and cared for.

It is based on the principle that we are all made of energy—ki—which runs through channels in the body known as the meridians. By using hands, elbows, knees, and feet, a shiatsu practitioner can move, change, and support ki, alleviating tension and promoting relaxation. Thus after treatment, people feel less stressed and are able to think more clearly and function more smoothly; the symptoms associated with a busy, adrenalin-filled life become less acute.

By developing an awareness of ki, anyone can apply, and benefit from, the techniques in this book, bringing joy and comfort both to the receiver of shiatsu and themselves.

why shiatsu?

In this age of technology and distant communication, shiatsu is a profound hands-on healing therapy, ideal for the stresses of modern life. You don't need any special equipment, just a willingness to learn and listen to the receiver's body. All you need to begin is a mat or futon, or even a chair if your receiver prefers. Shiatsu takes place fully clothed, so it is an excellent means of rediscovering the innocence of touch.

what is ki?

As we have seen, ki is the Japanese word for energy. Everything that lives,

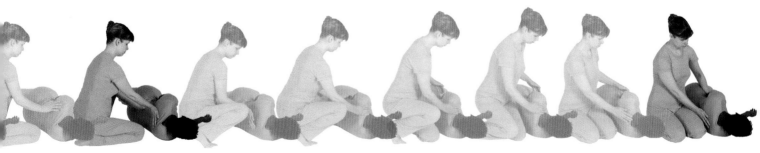

big or small, has or is ki. Trees, the earth, food, sea, sun, animals, and ourselves to name but a few all have ki. When ki is blocked or is at a low level, we feel unwell. Our minds fog over, we become depressed or angry, or our bodies start to grumble with the pain traditionally referred to as the "100 ills." When ki flows, we feel embodied, alive, vibrant, and able to face whatever challenges life may bring. Ki is never static, so we are always open to the possibility of change.

Shiatsu connects us to our ki. By supporting, holding, and listening to the receiver's body with an open heart, the giver and receiver cocreate opportunities for change.

the meridians

The meridians are channels of energy that run throughout the body. Each meridian represents a particular organ that has a physical, psychological, and spiritual significance. In shiatsu, because we work on the whole of the body, the meridians have been extended from the traditional Chinese system to do just that. This is known as the Masunaga system, after Shizuto Masunaga, who pioneered the Zen shiatsu system that is hugely popular today. In this book, points are used alongside Zen shiatsu meridians.

zen shiatsu

Zen shiatsu concentrates on treating the way the receiver feels at the present time, not what you may feel or think you should feel. It is based on the energetic theory of "kyo" and "jitsu," the opposite poles on which shiatsu treatment is based. Kyo qualities are often felt as cold, empty, tired, and lacking in life. Jitsu qualities are hot, tense, full, knotted, and hyperactive. The practitioner will support and "tonify" kyo areas in order to bring them to life. Tonification is a name for the holding and supporting techniques used to encourage ki to reinhabit kyo areas of the body. Thus the receiver is encouraged to reembody these empty, needy, or numb spaces. In jitsu areas, dispersal, rocking, and flowing techniques are used to encourage release from tension and stress and promote deep relaxation.

The practitioner will traditionally find out which meridians and areas of the body need treatment by hara diagnosis and a visual scan of the body, looking for areas that stand out as jitsu or hide kyo—for example, a receiver with shoulder problems may have one shoulder raised higher than the other. It is great practice just to watch people and see what you notice.

CUN MEASUREMENTS

Because everyone's body is different, meridians are located by a form of measurement called "cun," which measures the body by its own dimensions. Thus:

1 THUMB'S WIDTH = 1 CUN
2 FINGERS' WIDTH = 1.5 CUN
4 FINGERS' WIDTH = 3 CUN

the hara

The hara runs from below the ribcage to just above the pelvic bones in the abdominal area. In shiatsu, the hara is the diagnostic map of detailing the state of the receiver's body at the present time. All the meridians have a center here, which the practitioner will press and touch to feel for the most kyo and jitsu areas. Hara diagnosis is best taught by a teacher, but an awareness of the vulnerability and strength of the hara will make your initial shiatsu practice a much more healing experience.

For shiatsu givers, it is vital to build up this area in your own body as a source of power. Working on the floor demands specific skills of balance and a feeling of being connected to the ground. Coming from the hara means that you can work safely and draw on the earth for support.

yin yang theory

Yin yang is central to Chinese philosophy. Its symbol, the circle, which depicts wholeness, is made up of two halves divided by a flowing movement, both containing the seed of the other. Life force is expressed in this symbol.

Yin is the feminine, yielding, passive, resting form and Yang is the active, male, hot, solid side. Ever-shifting, they are interdependent energies, and everyone has their own relative balance of each.

When treating a receiver, it is important to judge what sort of shiatsu would benefit them most. For example, a receiver with big, strong, tight muscle structures is very yang and may not initially respond to yin holding and supportive techniques. Therefore, more active yang techniques and working positions should be used, such as the squatting and rocking practices shown throughout the book.

The yin principle of holding and stillness can then be used as the yang energy releases and energy shifts toward a deeper state of relaxation. This principle should be used with all receivers to ensure that they are neither over or underworked.

The interaction of these two forces and their relationship manifests as the five elements, which make up all things.

Yin yang theory is one of the fundamental principles of shiatsu. All practitioners must be aware of its importance when working on a receiver.

the five elements

The five element theory relates all energy and substance to one of the elements—fire, earth, metal (or air), water, and wood—and describes the growth of energy through the seasons, from winter to spring and summer and then autumn, encompassing the whole cycle of life. The table below illustrates the elemental qualities that exist in our bodies.

Remember, when you treat people with shiatsu, take a moment to consider whether they are more yin or yang in constitution. See which elements are strongest in their character and which need support. See if these are qualities you are drawn to work with and think about what this says about your own character.

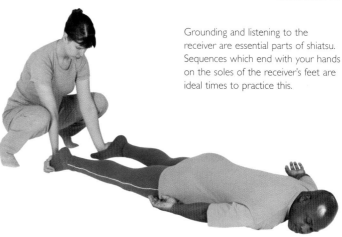

Grounding and listening to the receiver are essential parts of shiatsu. Sequences which end with your hands on the soles of the receiver's feet are ideal times to practice this.

ELEMENT	MERIDIAN	SEASON	FUNCTION	EMOTION	SOUND	COLOR	TASTE	SENSE	BODY TISSUE
water	kidney/bladder	winter	purification vitality	fear	groaning	blue/black	salty	hearing	bones
earth	spleen/stomach	transition	transformation	sympathy	singing	yellow	sweet	taste	flesh
fire	heart/ small intestines	summer	spiritual awareness assimilation	joy	laughter	red	bitter	speech	blood vessels
fire	heart protector triple heater	summer	communication protection	joy	laughter	red	bitter	speech	blood vessels
metal	lung/ large intestines	autumn	inspiration/ letting go	grief	weeping	white	spicy	smell	skin
wood	liver/gallbladder	spring	organisation	anger	shouting	green	sour	sight	muscle

meridian stretches

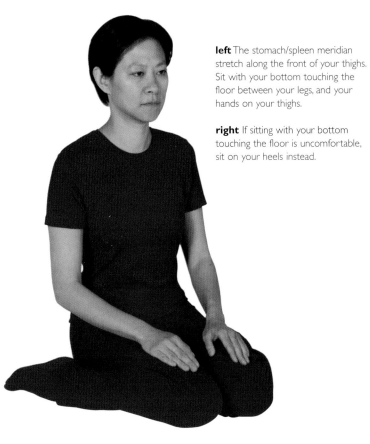

left The stomach/spleen meridian stretch along the front of your thighs. Sit with your bottom touching the floor between your legs, and your hands on your thighs.

right If sitting with your bottom touching the floor is uncomfortable, sit on your heels instead.

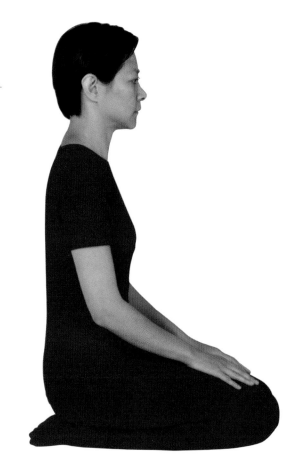

The following stretches illustrate where the meridians run and are good practice for both receivers and givers, as they open up the channels and stimulate the flow of ki. It is particularly good to be able to recommend specific stretches for the receiver—for example the gallbladder for inflexibility or the lungs and large intestine for depression—as a long list of stretches can be overwhelming.

Remember that as you practice these exercises, you should stretch forward on the outbreath or exhalation.

However, as a giver, it is important to take the time to work on yourself, learning to open up through stretching, yoga, t'ai chi, or meditation as this increases your sensitivity and allows you to maintain flexibility and build up your own ki.

below Gently lower yourself backward to further stretch the stomach/spleen meridian at the front of the thighs and the lower hara area on your torso.

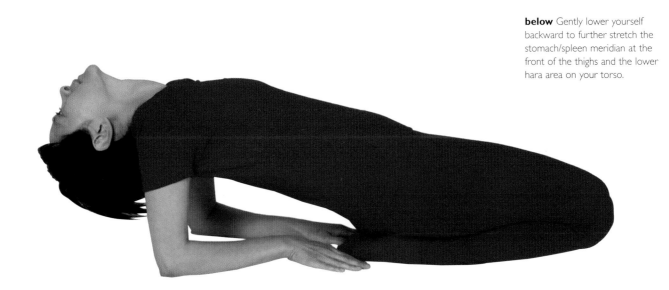

right The start of the
lung/large intestine stretch.
Clasp both hands together
behind your back, with feet
shoulder-width apart. This
opens the chest and improves
the lung intake of ki.
Then bend forward, lower
your head, and bring your
arms up over your head.
Keep your fingers straight up.
You should feel the stretch
in the back of each leg as
you bend forward.

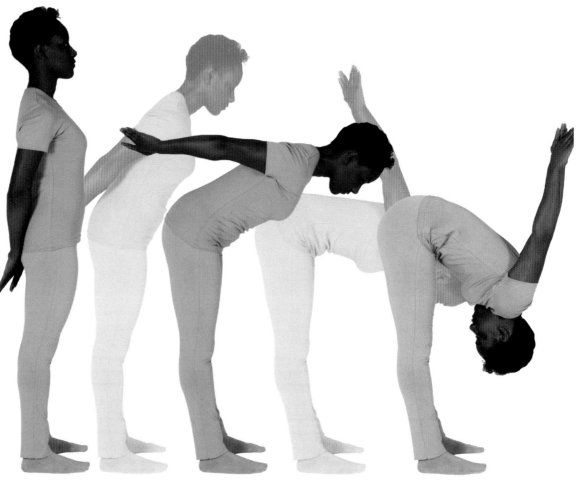

below The heart protector/triple heater stretch. Sit cross-legged, hands on opposite knees. Breathe out, stretch forward, and push your knees down. Feel the stretch in the sacrum and the lower edge of the outside of the thighs.

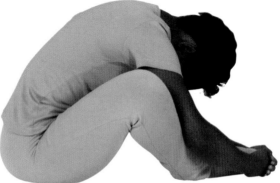

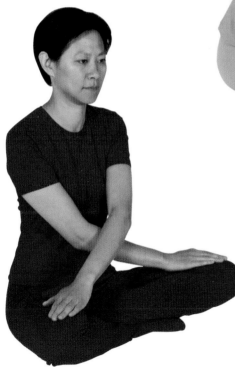

above Heart/small intestine stretch. Sit with the soles of your feet together, elbows on knees, and hands holding your feet. Allow yourself to lean foward on an out-breath.

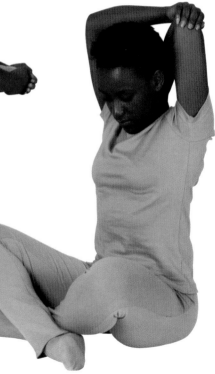

right The heart meridian stretch, along the lower edge of the inside of the upper arm. Sit cross-legged and pull one arm down behind your back, using your other hand. Grip your arm by the elbow. Repeat on the other side.

below The bladder/kidney meridian stretch. Sit on the floor upright, arms out in front of you, fingers outstretched. Reach forward toward your toes. Feel the stretch along the backs of your legs and your back. Try to get the whole of your back involved, rather than just focussing on touching your toes.

above The gallbladder/liver stretch, along the side of the body. Sit with your legs out straight, as wide apart as comfortable, with your hands clasped above your head. Don't overstretch as this will compromise the other compressed side of your body. Repeat on the other side.

the treatment

clothing

It is best for the receiver and giver to wear loose clothing made from natural fibers such as cotton so that ki can flow more freely. Close-fitting clothes were used in this book for the sake of visual clarity.

contraindications

The guidelines below list problems that beginners should avoid treating, although an experienced practitioner would be able to address them. If you have any doubts, always refer the receiver to an experienced shiatsu practitioner.

■ Fever, flu, or other acute illness where the body is fighting off invaders to its system.
■ High blood pressure
■ M.E. and other chronic fatique syndromes
■ First trimester of pregnancy
■ Heart disease
■ Cancer

Finally, avoid localized areas of swollen, raw, or inflamed skin, fractures, wounds, and scars from surgical operations, although treatment to the rest of the body can be very beneficial in helping to heal these conditions.

guidelines for receivers

As a practitioner, you need to let people know that they should:

■ Avoid eating a heavy meal on the day of treatment
■ Avoid alcohol
■ Try not to eat at least one hour before treatment
■ Enjoy!

SETTING FOR SHIATSU

It will give both you and your receiver more pleasure and a stronger base to work from if you treat each session as a ritual. For example:

■ Set up room, clean mat or futon and burn oils
■ Switch off phones and ensure you won't be disturbed
■ Bath or shower
■ Practice ki development exercises
■ Meditate
■ Lie down and wait for your client

Remember, shiatsu happens out of time, so create a space where healing can happen. Come from a place of respect, safety, and acceptance and from your hara and heart. Let go of all expectations and just listen, be, and enjoy.

shiatsu techniques

Once you have spoken to the receiver and observed their ki, you will want to begin. In order to give the best possible treatment, it is essential to practice and embody the following methods:

CRAWLING

POSTURE POSITIONS

MOTHER AND WORKING HAND CONNECTION

PERPENDICULAR PRESSURE

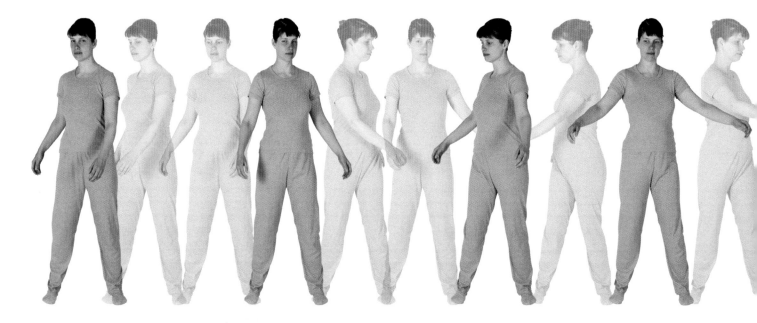

crawling

The basics of "crawling" will give you all the stability, connection, and grounding you need to give good shiatsu. Relax, breathe into your hara, and let the earth support you. Really let your weight "drop down" into the earth, relaxing any tension in your body. Keeping arms, shoulders, neck and thigh loose and moving with full self-awareness from your center of gravity will bring you into contact with the basic practice of shiatsu. In essence, you

Swing your arms from side to side. This allows ki to flow, ready for work. Swinging your arms also moves you out of your own boundary space, ready to meet the receiver.

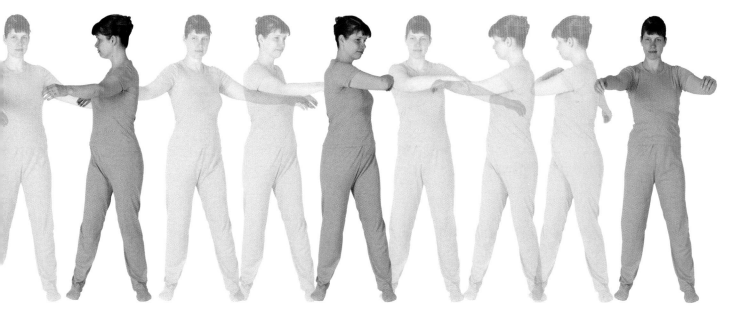

are aiming for the relaxation and control that you will observe in the movements of a cat. You can then experiment on a willing receiver by crawling around them, placing the palms of your hands on their body. You can see this skill translated into practice in the "catwalks" on pages 32–35.

Keep your hands relaxed and let them mold to the receiver's body. This will stop you worrying about what you "should" be doing and allows you to enter a deeper state of listening and balance, the perfect position for giving shiatsu from. Working from a deeper state of relaxation and sensitivity also ensures that we can feel whether a technique is opening the

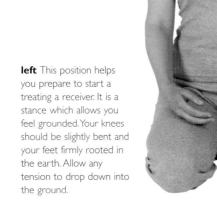

left This position helps you prepare to start a treating a receiver. It is a stance which allows you feel grounded. Your knees should be slightly bent and your feet firmly rooted in the earth. Allow any tension to drop down into the ground.

left The cezar position. Simply sit back on your heels. Use this position at the start of a treatment and when sitting by the side of the receiver.

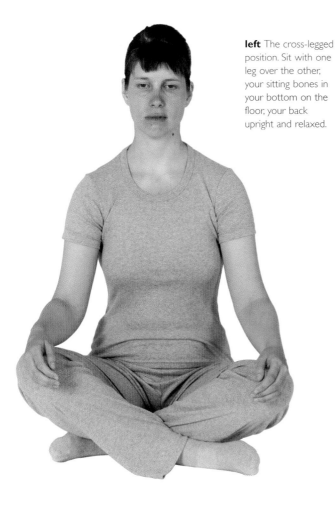

left The cross-legged position. Sit with one leg over the other, your sitting bones in your bottom on the floor, your back upright and relaxed.

receiver up or creating more tension. This is the starting point for sensing kyo and jitsu, and with time and practice, you will begin to feel these qualities as you crawl around the receiver.

posture positions

The best posture is to be relaxed and comfortable, with your breathing connected to your hara. Allow the earth to hold and support your weight and really let your center of gravity feel as if it is dropping down to a lower point. Ensure your hara is facing the area to be worked on for maximum results.

cezar and kneeling

Connect your legs, feet, and tailbone to the earth. Breathe into your hara and allow any tension to drop down, relaxing your shoulders.

cross-legged

Connect your perineum and legs to the earth. Breathe into the hara and allow any tension to drop down. This posture is perfect for more gentle yin treatment, where a yang way of working is not appropriate.

squatting

Relax your back and really let your weight drop down through your legs and feet into the ground. This is not an easy position to maintain and may initially feel physically demanding. It is worth practicing, however, because it gives a solidity and strength that will ultimately benefit the receiver.

It can also build up your ki if you take the time to practice positions by yourself and visualize your ki filling your hara with golden light that expands to fully support your stance. Allow your arms and shoulders to rest on this ki and your legs to be supported by this energetic strength.

As with all squatting positions, practice bouncing gently and try some side-to-side movements while in the squat to gain mobility and lightness.

Note these postures are very strong yang; so, if you like them, remember to keep your touch light and sensitive. This way your ki, rather than your body weight, moves the receiver's ki.

half-squatting

This involves squatting with one knee up, one knee down. Connect your

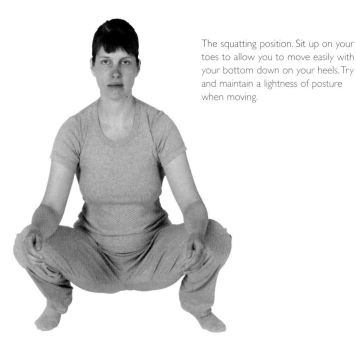

The squatting position. Sit up on your toes to allow you to move easily with your bottom down on your heels. Try and maintain a lightness of posture when moving.

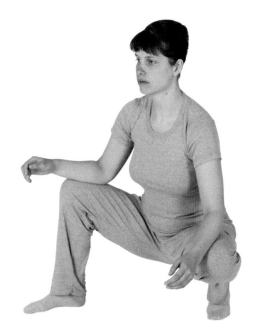

legs and feet to the earth, visualizing that you are really physically and energetically supported by the solid base it provides. Ensure that your hara is facing the area you are working on and keep a wide, comfortable base. The half-squat is a strong working position.

moving into treatment

Once you feel relaxed and at ease with these positions and their principles, you can experiment with touch.

mother and child hands

A connection between your two hands is essential to Zen shiatsu and gives the receiver complete support and the confidence to relax totally. Just as happens when a mother holds her child, one hand holds, supports, and provides stillness, while the other works down the body, responding to kyo and jitsu. Together, they are one, energetically connected to each other and the receiver at all times.

Traditionally, the mother hand is the most important of the two, as it provides the support necessary for the receiver to relax and a place of stillness for the giver to imbibe and listen to the effects of the treatment. However,

The mother and child hands. You can sit cross-legged if you wish as an alternative to working in the cezar position. This is a more yin way of working and is good for practicing connecting the mother and child hands.

the two hands work as one and the giver should develop an awareness of their connection at all times. Think of how odd a one-armed hug feels and you'll see exactly why one-handed shiatsu is not quite as satisfying. Thus, as far as physically possible, the two hands should never leave the body. When you have to move them, connect with your "intention" to support the receiver. Intention means being completely focussed on the client and not letting your mind wander. It also involves listening to the receiver's body with your hands and feelings and visualizing a depth of connection.

As an exercise, practice crawling on the receiver with mother and child hands, the mother hand on the hara and the child hand working down the receiver's legs.

penetration and perpendicular pressure

Using the positions and postures so far described, it should be apparent that any work on the meridian points (tsubos) comes from a place of deep relaxation rather than physical force. There are times when a shiatsu treatment needs to be deep. This depth does not come from applying extra force with the muscles but from a whole body connection of which the receiver is a part. Place arms, hands, or thumbs perpendicular to the surface of the body. Breathe deeply and imagine your ki travelling through the receiver to the earth below. Deep connection comes from focus, working at the correct angle (your hands should work perpendicular to the receiver's body), listening, and awareness—all centered in the hara. Attempting to use physical pressure instead will cause a defensive reaction in the receiver's ki,

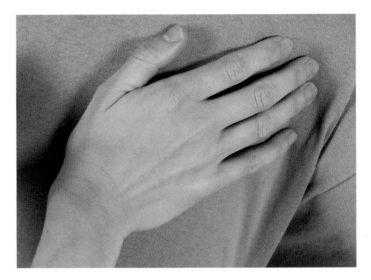

Palming is usually carried out by moving you hand in a "wave" motion, starting with the heel of the hand and rolling on to the fingers.

blocking ki connection. Too much pressure does not feel safe.

However, static, energetically supportive work is particularly effective in encouraging ki to kyo areas, so it is an essential skill to develop. Tsubos in particular benefit from perpendicular pressure because of their structure, which is often likened to a jar with a narrow neck. When the "neck" is

penetrated perpendicularly, it leads into the space below, occupied by the receiver's ki. A giver who doesn't access this space will simply be brushing the surface where jitsu can be contacted, but the depths of kyo will never be addressed.

palming

With this powerful technique, your hands mold to the receiver's body. From a relaxed, earthed position, this is a good place to start a treatment, as you can practice two-handed connection and scan for kyo and jitsu areas.

Palming techniques can involve the use of both hands, generating a feeling of connectivity between them as they work on the receiver.

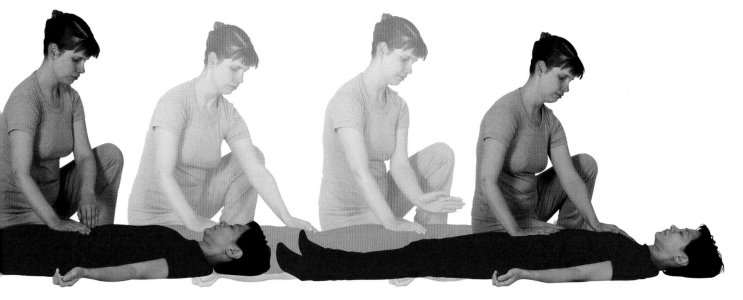

Thumbing: keep your thumb straight and support it with your hand, which should be held in a loose fist. This ensures you won't hurt your thumb.

Remember always to work perpendicular to the meridian—don't work on meridians from any other angle.

thumbs

Thumbing is the most characteristic shiatsu technique and is suitable for applying firm pressure and listening to the receiver's ki. It should be supported by the rest of the hand, as in the picture, in order to prevent stress and strain to the joints. The thumb should also be kept as straight as possible in order to avoid any damage. Again, it is important to achieve a two-handed connection, so you can either use two thumbs together or one thumb and one hand so that the receiver does not have the feeling of being poked.

fingertips

Finger pressure is not as physically penetrating as thumb work, but good ki penetration can still be achieved by using the fingers simultaneously. As you work, the thumb should be relaxed and the fingers strong. Breathe into your hara and feel the movement come through the elbow rather than the wrist.

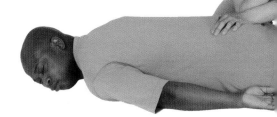

elbows

Practice working with your elbows with care, as elbow pressure can be very strong and forceful. Only use it after you feel comfortable with the other techniques and are ready to move on. As always, ensure you are working from your hara and in a comfortable working posture. Allow yourself to be relaxed and use the point of your elbow to work with. This gives deep penetration. Keep your mother hand or arm in place to track your receiver's reactions. Do not use elbows in bony or weak areas of the body. Save them for the more robust regions—the buttocks, backs, and thighs.

Elbows are powerful tools, so they must be used with care. Be sure to listen to the receiver if you are working in this way.

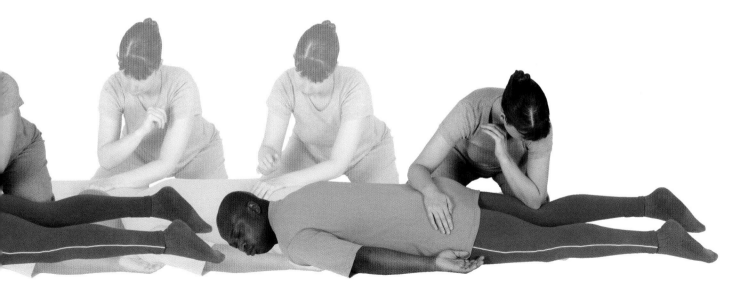

endings

Ending the treatment is a sensitive time. The receiver may have been through any number of emotional experiences you may not be aware of. Allow them a short time to share their thoughts and feeling if they wish, but try to avoid a doctor-style analysis. Remember, shiatsu happens in a different time frame to that which governs everyday life. Healing is empowerment, so only share knowledge that you feel will truly empower your receiver. Once the receiver has left, take a little time to come back to yourself. Enjoy.

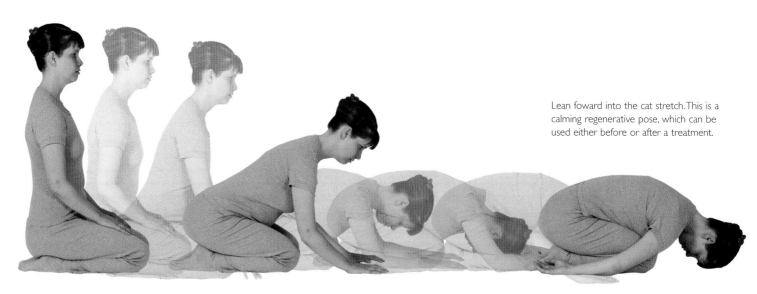

Lean foward into the cat stretch. This is a calming regenerative pose, which can be used either before or after a treatment.

go with the flow

The special Flowmotion images used in this book have been created to show every stage of the subtle processes of connection involved in shiatsu, and not just isolated highlights. Each shiatsu sequence is shown across the page from left to right, demonstrating how the move progresses safely and effectively for both giver and receiver, and is fully explained with step-by-step captions. Below this, another layer of information in the timeline breaks the move into its various key stages, with instructions for "breathing," "earthing," "listening," "connecting," and so on. The symbols in the timeline also include instructions for when to pause and hold a position and when to move seamlessly from one stage to the next.

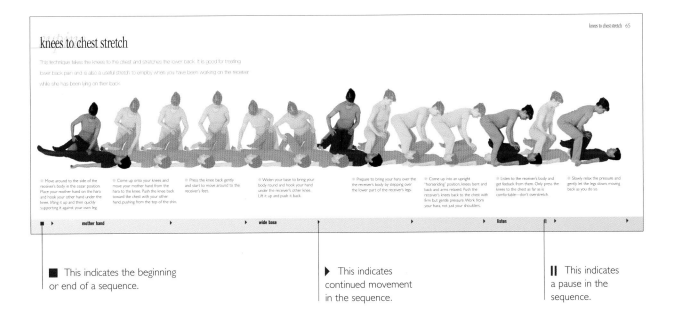

knees to chest stretch

This technique takes the knees to the chest and stretches the lower back. It is good for treating lower back pain and is also a useful stretch to employ when you have been working on the receiver while she has been lying on their back.

■ This indicates the beginning or end of a sequence.

▶ This indicates continued movement in the sequence.

❙❙ This indicates a pause in the sequence.

prone

connecting and opening stretches

First contact is very important in shiatsu. Recognizing and developing the ability to connect with both yourself and the receiver is a theme that runs throughout the practice of this ancient art.

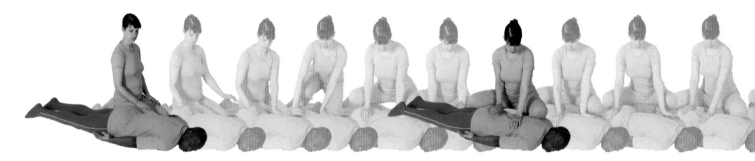

● Shiatsu is all about feeling connected. Sit back on your heels, with your back upright but relaxed. This is the "cezar" position. The receiver lies face down, arms by sides. Place one hand on the sacrum.

● Open up the receiver's back, especially the area around the sacrum and the kidneys, with the palms of your hands, using a relaxed padding motion. Relax and practice listening for differences in ki.

● Move into a squat position so you can easily access the back without having to compromise your own posture. Your hara should be facing the receiver's back and be the center you are working from.

● As you work up and down the back, move your hips from side to side to face the part of the back you are working on. Allow your movement to come from your hara.

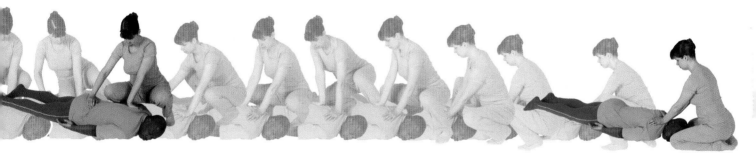

● Your hands should continue to work around the back. This padding motion opens up the back and is preparatory work.

● Start to move from the back, working around to the top of the head. Your posture should remain the same—back loose and shoulders relaxed—as you continue to pad.

● Listen to what your hands are telling you. Try to stay aware of the different responses the receiver's body is giving you and focus on your own quality of touch.

● When you have worked your way around to the head, sit back in the cezar position, keeping a wide base. Do not let your legs come too close to the receiver's head. Work from your hara rather than your shoulders.

▶ **relax** ▶   ▶ **wide base** ▶

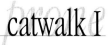# catwalk I

The catwalk opens up the main meridian, known as the bladder meridian, down the back.

This technique is great for everyone as it relaxes the autonomic nervous system. When doing

the catwalk, attempt to mimic the feline rhythm of a cat as it moves.

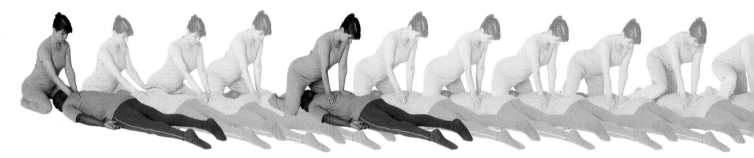

● Start in the cezar position and breathe to develop a feeling of being earthed. Place your hands either side of the receiver's spine, 1.5 cun from the middle of the spine, just below the neck. Tune into the receiver's ki.

● Lift one hand and place it further down the spine and then repeat with the other hand. Movement comes from the hara and should be feline-like rather than just lifting and dropping the hand.

● Start to bring your weight up as you move onto your knees. Your center of gravity should still be low in your hara.

● As you continue to "walk" down the spine, start to bring one knee up. Keep your shoulders relaxed and make a conscious effort to breathe and be aware of your hara.

▶ **connect and earth** ▶ **breathe** ▶ ▶

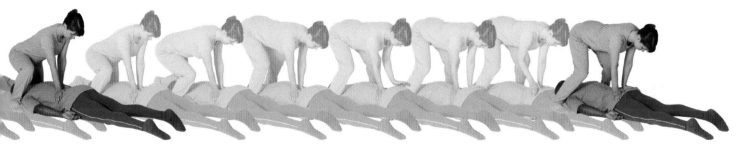

● As you continue to become more upright, move your weight slightly from side to side as your hands walk one at a time down the back. Stay in hara.

● Keep your knees bent, so there is no pressure on your lower back, and let your back stay straight but loose.

● Visualize your energy coming down your arms from your hara. The looser and more relaxed you are, the better.

● Your hands should go all the way down to the receiver's sacrum and finish side by side.

stay in hara ▶ ▶ **relax** ▶ ▶

catwalk II

The second part of the catwalk continues to open the bladder meridian and back. Bear in mind the physical build of the receiver when applying pressure with your hands; small-framed people need to be worked on less vigorously. This ties in with listening to the receiver's body—an essential ingredient of shiatsu.

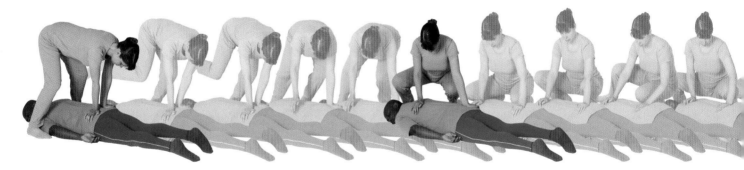

● With your knees bent, relax into an earthed position. Take your weight on your feet and connect to the receiver's ki. Place your hands on the edge of the receiver's sacrum, stretching it out.

● Step outside the receiver's head toward a semi-squat position. Keep in hara to stay balanced.

● Place one hand on the edge of the sacrum, the other in line with the scapula, but just below it. Your hands, the "mother and child", should be on opposite sides of the spine. This works on the kidney meridian.

● Keeping the hara central, start to move your hands over the receiver's body toward the reverse of the previous hand position. Avoid just jumping to the new position. This completes the stretch.

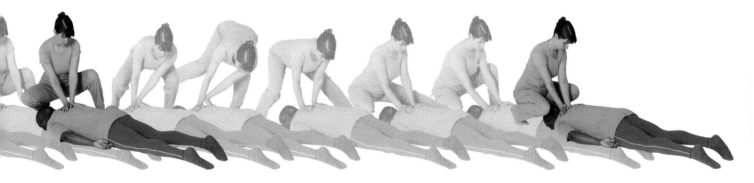

● Gently rock your weight from side to side as you work your hands and return to the upper back area.

● As you work your way around the receiver's head, come up out of the squatting position and adopt a wide stance, with both legs bent and your back loose. Your hands should be 1.5 cun from the middle of the spine.

● Moving one leg at a time, come back down into a squat as your body clears the receiver's head. Keep your hands in the upper back area.

● Tune into the receiver's ki. This will tell you how long to maintain the pressure with your hands.

▶   ▶ **relax**   ▶   ▶

thumb down bladder meridian

This technique involves working with your thumbs to hit "yu" points along the back. Yu points are diagnostic areas that relate to the body's main organs. Remember to work with a straight thumb, using the point—rather than the pad—of your thumb. Use your first finger and hand, held as a loosely closed fist, for support.

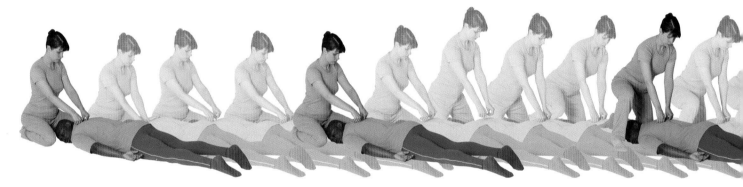

In the cezar position, place your thumbs 1.5 cun from the center of the spine, a little below the top of the shoulder blades (scapula). This is on the border of the third thoracic vertebra and is the lung yu point.

Bringing in pressure gradually, work down either side of the spine in a straight line. The next yu point is outside the next vertebra down and is the heart protector point.

Come up onto your knees, but keep your weight low in your hara. Listen to the feedback from the receiver's body.

Switch off from any conscious thought and allow your awareness of the receiver's body to come through the points of your thumbs.

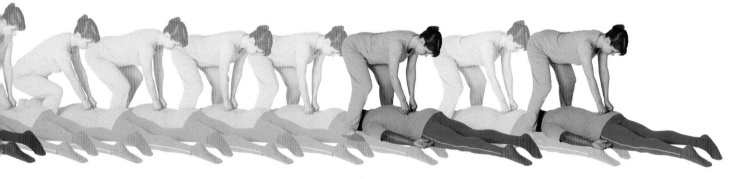

◉ Continue to work down the spine, keeping your thumbs straight. Pause and keep pressure on points where you feel little feedback from the receiver's body. This may be kyo, so listen carefully.

◉ As you work along the length of the spine, you will work yu points for the heart, diaphragm, liver, gallbladder, and spleen.

◉ Lower down the spine, you will work yu points for the stomach, triple heater, kidneys, and large intestine.

◉ As you come to the sacrum, the first set of indentations on either side of the spine are the yu points for the small intestine. The second set of indentations are yu points for the bladder. Enjoy finding them.

▶   ▶   **relax**   ▶   ▶

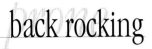

back rocking

Back rocking releases tension and encourages ki to flow more freely. This technique should not
be practiced on someone with very low ki, as it would completely disperse any remaining energy.
Back rocking can also be used as a starting point instead of the catwalk.

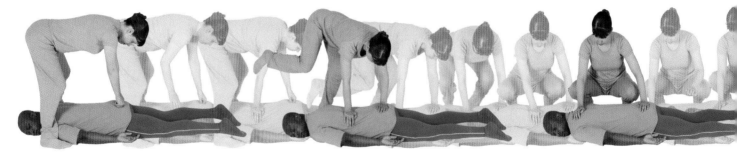

● Continuing from the previous page,
here you connect and prepare to
change over from one technique to
the next. Make sure you are grounded
before the next movement.

● Change from using your thumbs to
using your palms. Place one hand on
the sacrum and the other on the
middle of the back.

● Step over the receiver's head,
keeping centered in your hara. Come
down into a squat position beside
the receiver.

● In the squat position, hold the
sacrum with one hand and move the
other to the top of the back, level
with the scapula, on the far side of the
spine. Tune in to the receiver.

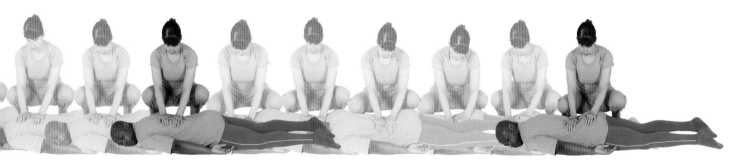

● Move the hand on the sacrum to rest beside the hand at the top of the back. Using the heels of the hands, move backward and forward from your hara, in a rocking motion.

● As you rock, gradually work your hands down the far side of the receiver's back. This method of working from the top of the body down is a principle of zen shiatsu.

● Finish off working on the back area on the sacrum.

● When you have completed the technique, turn around and repeat the process on the other side.

listen ▶ ▶ ▶ ▶

leg rocking

Leg rocking continues the theme started in back rocking but this time, as the name suggests, the technique is carried on to the legs. Leg rocking is good for dispersing jitsu.

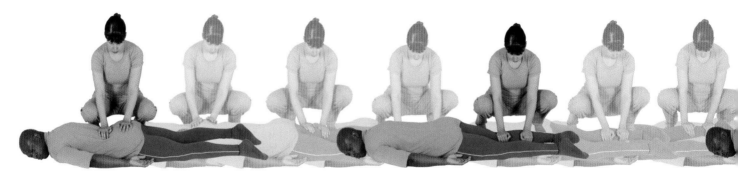

⬤ Continuing from the sacrum, the finishing point of the back-rocking technique, bring your hands down onto the buttocks and continue with the rocking motion. Remember to retain your own posture.

⬤ Maintain a wide, stable base and start to work your hands down the leg. It is important to be earthed— remember that your movements are initiated from your hara.

⬤ Let your hands wrap around the contours of the leg as you rock backward and forward. Your movement comes through the heels of your hands.

⬤ Continue to work down the leg to the calf. Your back should be loose and your shoulders relaxed.

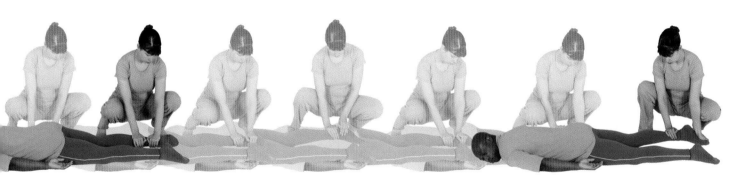

● When you reach the ankle, your hands can completely surround this narrow part of the leg. Work on the ankle using a wave motion from the heel of the hand to the fingertips.

● To keep your hara central to where you are working, shift your weight slightly from side to side as necessary.

● As you reach the foot, you are approaching a major grounding point. One hand should be around the ankle, the other with the palm on the top third of the foot in the center of the sole.

● The hand on the sole of the foot is on a major point on the kidney meridian (kidney 1) as well as a major grounding point.

bent-knee stretch

This move stretches the quadrucep, the muscle on the front of the thigh. In shiatsu, this muscle lies on the spleen meridian. This a very effective technique for grounding the receiver, but should be used with caution or not at all if the receiver suffers from lower back pain.

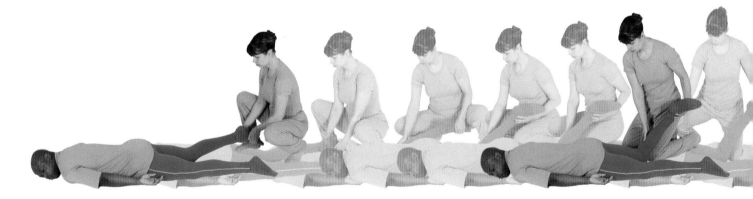

In a half-squat position, place your hands under the receiver's foot and take a firm but loose grip.

Gripping the foot, give it a little shake to relieve any tension in the leg. This also lets the receiver know that the stretch is about to start.

Lifting the foot up into the stretch, bring one hand onto the shin and move your own position to be outside the receiver's leg. This centers your hara on the area of activity.

Keep one hand under the foot, relaxed but supportive. Check with the receiver that the stretch in the front of the thigh is not becoming uncomfortable.

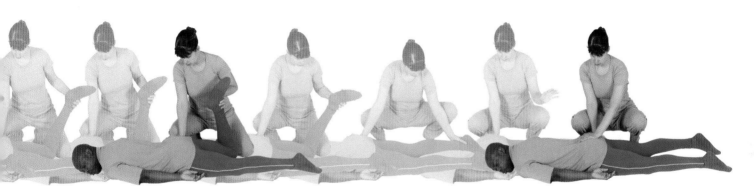

● Bring one hand up to the edge of the buttock. This allows you to listen to the receiver's body. Press down slightly on this point as well. This stops the lower back from curving too much during the stretch.

● Move from this low position to a higher semi-squat one. This allows you to be closer to the receiver's body and lets you work directly over it. It also keeps your hara centered to the movement of the stretch.

● With one hand on the edge of the buttock, move the other one to the outside of the ankle. Lower the leg to reverse the stretch and open up the back of the limb. Your own stance should move into an open squat.

● Closing your stance slightly, move your hand from the ankle to the sacrum. This is a point of stillness.

listen ▶ **stay in hara** ▶ **stillness** ‖

elbows over buttocks and thighs

This technique is good for loosening tight muscle structures. However, the elbows are capable of exerting considerable power, so start contact gently and use it judiciously, remembering to work from your hara. Your elbows are useful for working on tight, jitsu areas.

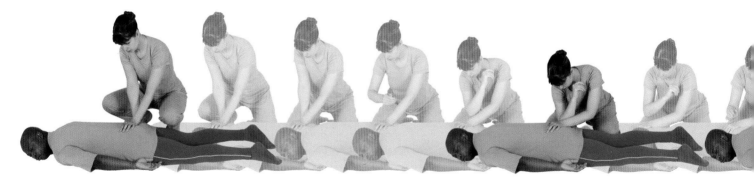

● Start from a point of stillness, with your hands on the receiver's sacrum. Start padding around the area to loosen up this region of the back and prepare it for elbow work. Remember to breathe.

● Remember to work from your hara. It is all too easy to work just from your shoulders.

● Apply pressure to the buttocks with the point of your elbow. You will have to bend your arm to do this. The point of the elbow is used for accuracy and increased depth of treatment.

● Keep your mother hand in the strong supportive position on the sacrum. This is your listening hand.

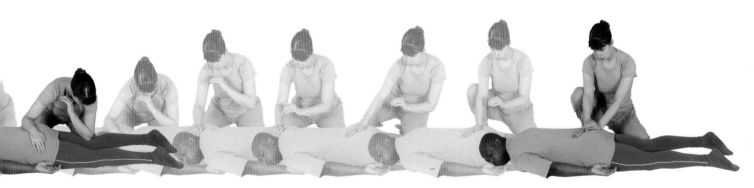

● As you work down the back of the thigh, swap arms and use your right forearm for support. This enables you to come down low without twisting and compromising your body position.

● Try to work down the center of the leg, the bladder meridian. Only go as far as the knee and ask the receiver for feedback as you work.

● Change from using your forearm for support to using only your hand, which should be returned to the sacrum. Keep in contact with the receiver's body as you make this movement.

● Move your other hand back up the body and shift into a semi-squat stance as you do so. Place this hand next to the one on the sacrum.

▶   ▶   ▶   **stillness**   ■

thumb down thigh & calves bladder meridian

This technique works the bladder meridian, which relaxes the autonomic nervous system.

It is a very useful method of treating all types of nervous disorders.

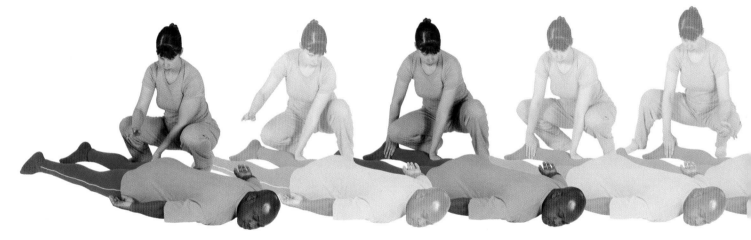

● Continuing from the position on the previous page, ground and listen to the receiver. Connect your mother hand to the receiver's sacrum, with the child hand ready to move down the leg.

● From the squat position, prepare to start thumbing. Keep your thumb straight, supported by your index finger, and the rest of your hand held in a loose fist.

● Start to work down the middle of the back of the receiver's leg with your thumb, listening for kyo and jitsu.

● As you work down the back of the leg, keep as wide a base as possible. Your hara should be facing the area you are working on.

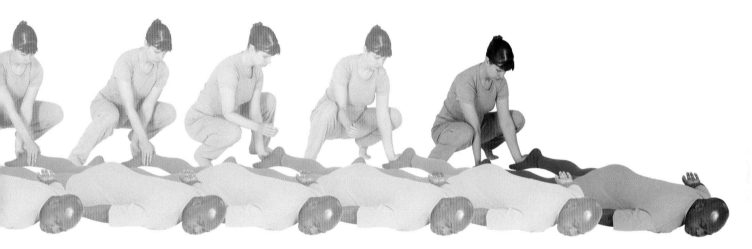

● Work down towards the receiver's calves, always keeping in ki contact as you move. Move your mother hand down behind the knee as the child hand works down the middle of the calf.

● Move your body around to face the soles of the receiver's feet. Hold one ankle with your mother hand in a "dragon's claw" by pressing either side of the achilles tendon. Palm down the middle of the foot with your child hand.

● As an alternative to palming, press down the outside edge of the foot instead, finishing at the end of the outside edge of the little toenail. This the end of the bladder meridian.

● Move your hands to a position two-thirds down the middle of the foot. Your palms should now be on kidney 1. Ground and listen.

footshake & holding

The footshake encourages ki to flow down the legs and releases any energy held in the sacrum and lower back. Avoid using this technique if the receiver has back problems.

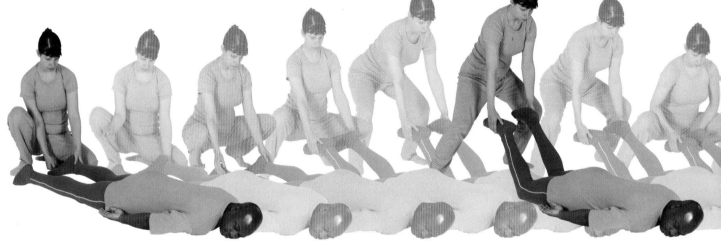

In a half-squat position, place one hand on the ankle and the other on the lower third of the foot. Make sure you are grounded and that your hara is earthed.

Come up into a full squat and place one hand on each ankle, near the heel.

Raise yourself into a more upright position, lifting the receiver's legs as you do so. Keep your knees bent and your back relaxed. It is important to visualize your hara connecting directly to the ground.

Cradling the receiver's feet near the ankles, swing the legs from side to side. Listen to the receiver's body as you move. Be sure you get a firm grip of the feet—socks can be slippery.

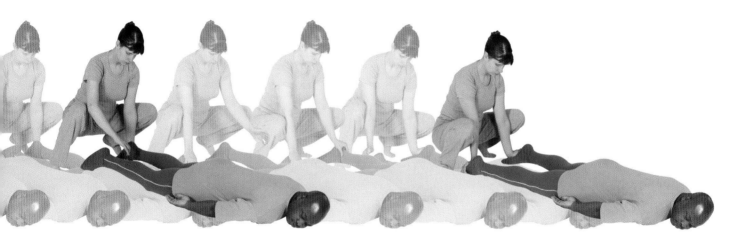

● Come back down into a squat, lowering the receiver's legs as you do so. Keep rocking the legs from side to side on the way down. Take care to let the legs down carefully.

● When moving your hands over the receiver's feet and ankles, move one hand only at a time. This makes sure contact is never lost with the receiver and maintains intention of ki contact.

● Stay in this earthed, squatting position as you approach the end of the technique.

● Place your hands on the bottom two-thirds of each foot, with your fingers out to the sides. This is an important grounding point for the receiver and is called kidney I.

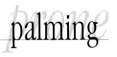

palming

Palming is a basic shiatsu concept. It involves making contact with the receiver and seeing what you can feel, listening for kyo and jitsu. It follows the motion of a baby crawling.

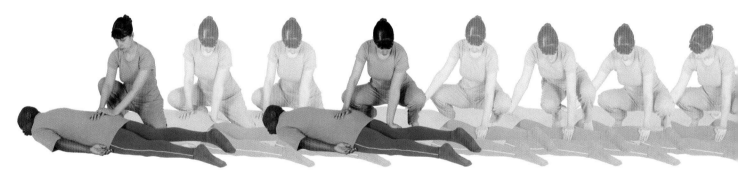

● In a half-squat position, place one hand on the sacrum and the other next to it. Make sure you are earthed and tuned in to the receiver—be receptive to what you feel.

● With one hand on the sacrum, start to palm down one leg with the other hand. Keep your palming hand relaxed, but make firm contact with the heel of the hand. Allow the rest of the hand and fingers to curl around the leg.

● Work down the center of the leg, keeping your fingers on the outside when in the thigh area to avoid touching the groin. Listen with your mother hand (on the sacrum) and move the child hand (palming) in response.

● Turn your hand around so your fingers are on the inside of the leg when you get below the knee.

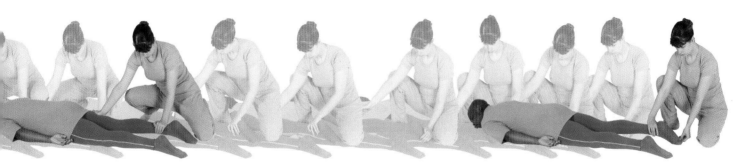

● As your child hand reaches the bottom of the leg, move the mother hand further down the thigh. Keep in ki contact as well as in physical contact.

● Continue to move your mother hand down the leg. Place your child hand on the lower two-thirds of the sole of the foot on kidney 1. Notice that the child hand now becomes the supporting hand.

● Bring your mother hand down to the ankle. In a half-squat, pull on each of the toes with your child hand.

● Finally, come to a point of earthed stillness. Repeat on the other leg, starting at "leg rocking" on pages 40–41.

supine

connect to earth, clockface on hara

In shiatsu, the hara is the center of the body. The technique demonstrated here allows you to experience working with the hara and become receptive to what the receiver is feeling.

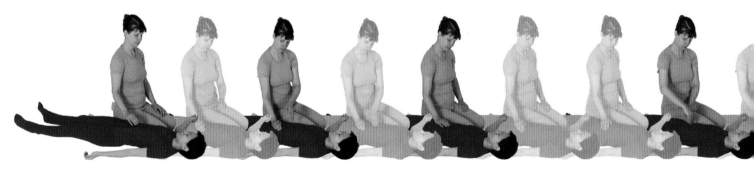

● Sit in the cezar position and make sure you are really grounded. With one hand resting on the receiver's lower abdomen, tune into their breathing. Breathe easily yourself and be ready to meet the receiver's ki.

● Pause for a moment and let the receiver get used to your hand being on their abdomen.

● Start to move your hand around their abdomen in a clockwise direction.

● Bring your other hand on and move around the clockface, one hand following the other, using your fingertips,

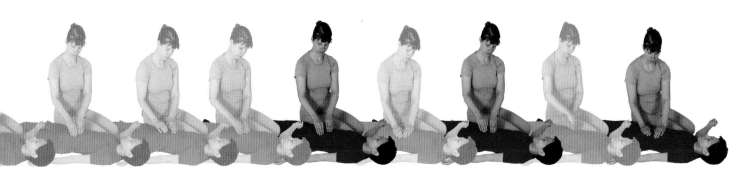

⬤ Feel for different qualities of ki and be guided by what you feel. Don't work too deep — remember that the hara is an intimate space.

⬤ If it is kyo, work deeper, but again be aware of the sensitivity of the area you are working on.

⬤ Finish with your mother hand on the hara. This gives the receiver a feeling of being held energetically and lets them relax to a deeper level.

⬤ Your child hand finishes at the top of the hara. Feel the connection between your hands.

rocking in hara & down legs

Rocking down the legs relaxes the abdominal organs and gives the receiver a feeling of awareness about their own body. Try to get a wave motion going in your hands over the receiver's hara.

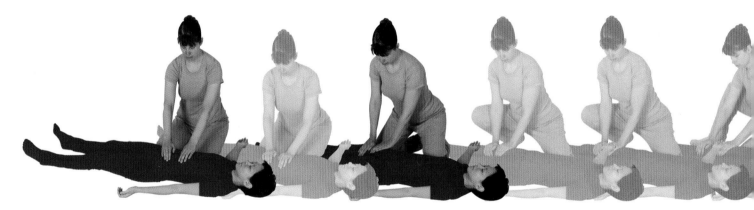

● Get into a half-raised cezar position, with as broad a base as possible. Feel grounded and relax your shoulders and your hands. The wave motion for this technique involves pushing with the palms, then pulling back with the fingertips.

● Move your hands to the top of the leg and start to work down, using the wave motion in your hands, and rocking as you do so. Avoid starting too far up on the thigh as this can be intrusive for the receiver.

● In a kneeling position, move down the leg. Keep grounded and as close to the body as is comfortable. This avoids overstretching.

● Work down the leg toward the ankle, turning your body to face the area you are working on as you go. You will have to adopt a semi-squatting position. Remember to breathe deeply and relax.

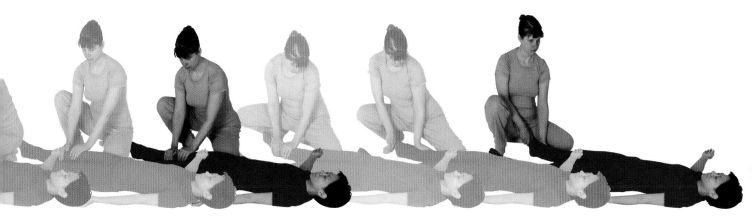

● When you reach the foot, move from your position at the side of the receiver's body to a position at the foot so your hara is directly facing the receiver's opposite shoulder.

● Change hand positions so that one hand is cradling the ankle and the other is on the sole of the foot, holding it near the ball. Keep the rocking motion going.

● Take the rocking motion into the toes.

● Rock each toe in turn and then pull on all toes together.

breathe   ▶   **rock**   ▶   ▶   ■

leg rotation keeping hand on hara

Leg rotations pivot around the hip, opening up it and the groin area. They also encourage flexibility and increase the flow of ki.

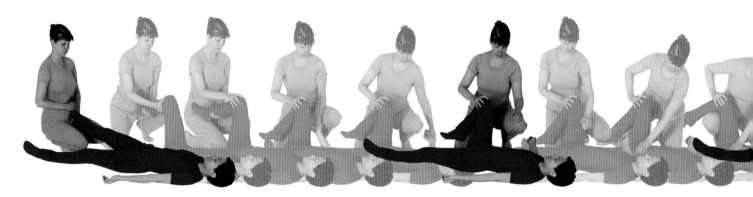

● From a grounded cezar position, hold one of the receiver's feet. With one hand on the top of the foot and the other supporting the ankle, press the sole against your hara. This is a point of stillness.

● Come up into a semi-squat, supporting the leg with your own raised leg and the hand under the ankle. Also, support it with your hara. Place your other hand on the knee.

● Move the receiver's arm out to the side to make room for you to come beside them. Get as close as possible to the receiver to give them good support.

● Place one hand on the receiver's hara. This is the listening hand. As you reach down, shift your weight to lower one knee and raise the other.

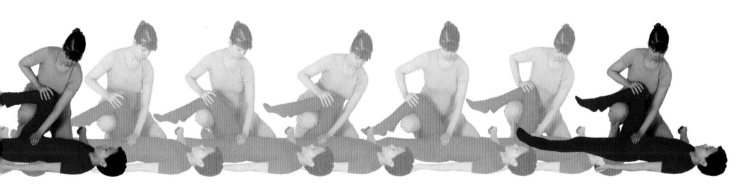

● Place the receiver's leg over your raised knee and start to rotate it in small, clockwise circles. You will need to rotate with them. Keep your hand on their hara and listen. Give their leg lots of support with your own.

● Avoid overrotating the receiver's leg. The rotation should be challenging but comfortable. Make small circles first, and then increase to larger ones.

● Then repeat the technique, rotating the leg the other way in an counterclockwise direction.

● When you have completed rotations in both directions, come to a point of stillness before the next stage.

listen ▶ ▶ **repeat** ▶ **breathe** ▶

leg stretch & palming

The leg stretch extends the thigh muscle. It opens up the spleen meridian and is a useful technique to help you become grounded.

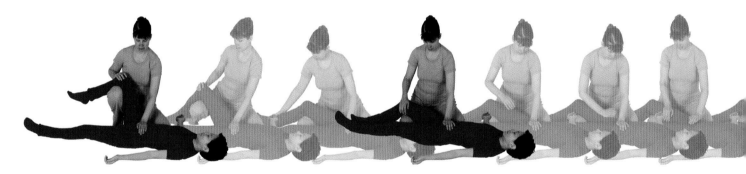

● Prepare to move into the leg stretch. Drop your supporting leg and move the knee out to the side to form a wide base, supporting the receiver's leg as you move.

● Open out the receiver's leg to the side, as far as is comfortable. The big toe on the stretched leg should rest against the ankle of the other leg. Remember to keep the stretched leg supported with your own leg.

● Keep your mother hand on the hara. Open the stretched leg further with the other hand on the inside of the knee. Keep your back relaxed and remember to breathe.

● Move the hand on the knee to the top of the thigh and start to palm down the leg toward the knee. Turn your hand so your fingers are on the outside of the leg while working on the upper thigh.

▶ **breathe** ▶ **support** ▶ **breathe** ▶

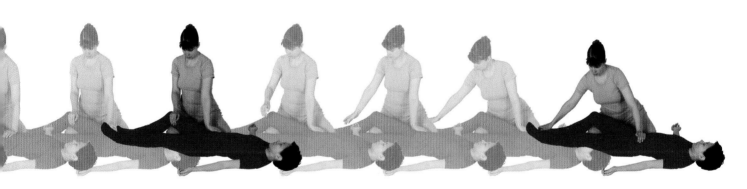

● The palming motion should involve pressing with the heel of the hand, then pulling back with the fingers. Work down the inside edge of the thigh muscle, which will appear down the center of the leg because the leg is stretched open,

● Move the hand on the receiver's hara to the top of the thigh where the thigh muscle joins the hip.

● Continue to work down the leg. When you reach the lower leg, palm down the inside of the shin bone to the foot. Return the hand on the hip flexor meridian to the receiver's hara.

● When you reach the foot, palm down the inside of the foot. Continue down the edge of the big toe. This is the end point of the meridian.

hara ankle rotation

Ankle rotations follow the same principles as hip rotation. This technique loosens up the ankle tendons and unwinds the whole body. It ensures the receiver feels wonderfully held and supported.

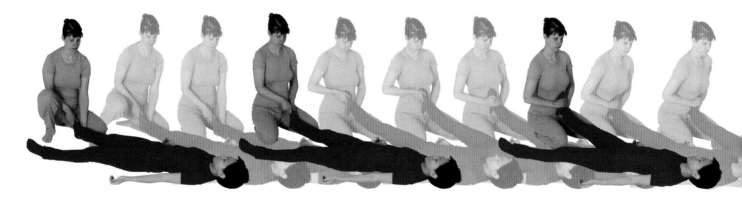

● In a semi-squat position, support the ankle with one hand and place the other hand on top of the foot. This makes contact with the receiver.

● Kneeling in the cezar position, make as wide a base as possible as you start to lift the foot.

● Bring the receiver's foot up to your hara. It should fit snugly to create a strong connection between you and the receiver.

● Start to rotate the ankle slowly by rotating your upper body from the hips. Hold the foot firmly against your hara and tune in to the receiver. This starts to unwind and open the ankle.

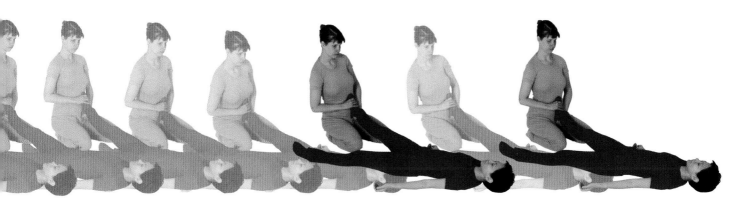

● Once you have completed the
rotations in one direction, repeat them
in the other direction.

● Make sure that you hold the
receiver's foot near the top, with the
thumb pressed against the sole.

● Keep your arms and back relaxed
and try to work from your hara.

● Although this is a gentle technique,
there is still lots of movement, so finish
with a point of stillness.

▶ **listen** ▶ ▶ ■

knees to chest stretch

This technique takes the knees to the chest and stretches the lower back. It is good for treating lower back pain and is also a useful stretch to employ when you have been working on the receiver while she has been lying on their back.

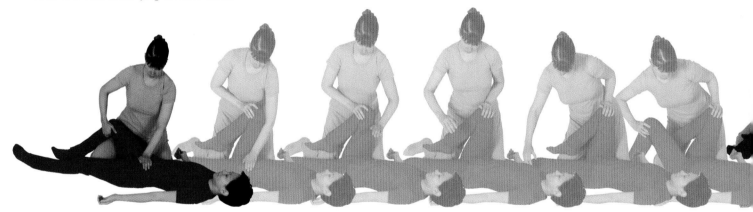

● Move around to the side of the receiver's body in the cezar position. Place your mother hand on the hara and hook your other hand under the knee, lifting it up and then quickly supporting it against your own leg.

● Come up onto your knees and move your mother hand from the hara to the knee. Push the knee back toward the chest with your other hand, pushing from the top of the shin.

● Press the knee back gently and start to move around to the receiver's feet.

● Widen your base to bring your body round and hook your hand under the receiver's other knee. Lift it up and push it back.

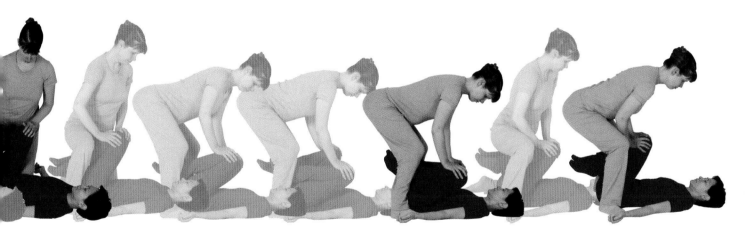

● Prepare to bring your hara over the the receiver's body by stepping over the lower part of the receiver's legs.

● Come up into an upright "horseriding" position, knees bent and back and arms relaxed. Push the receiver's knees back to the chest with firm but gentle pressure. Work from your hara, not just your shoulders.

● Listen to the receiver's body and get feeback from them. Only press the knees to the chest as far as is comfortable—don't overstretch.

● Slowly relax the pressure and gently let the legs down, moving back as you do so.

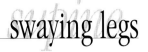

swaying legs

Working on the legs by swaying them loosens up the connection between the lower back, the sacrum, and the legs. It is a useful technique for hip and sacrum problems.

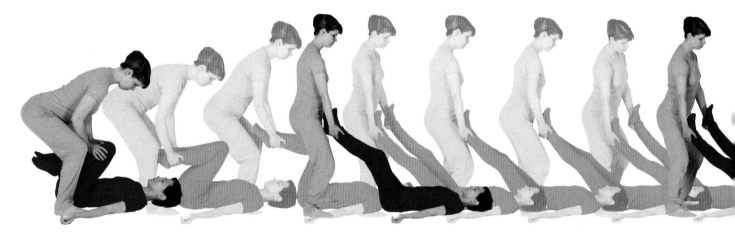

● Continuing from the position on the previous page, make sure you are grounded and breathe deeply.

● Move back slightly, rising as you do so. Slide your hands back to just above the receiver's ankles and let the receiver's legs begin to straighten out.

● Stand almost upright, but with bent legs, solidly grounded. Allow the weight of the receiver's legs to fall into your hands rather than trying to exert a strong grip on them. If you stay relaxed, the receiver will do the same.

● Sway the legs from side to side in a fluid movement. Make sure the receiver's legs are not locked straight.

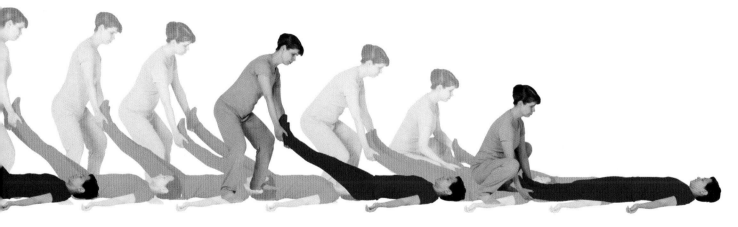

● Allow your knees to bend and let your body start to come down toward the ground. Keep swaying the receiver's legs as you come down. Remember not to let the receiver's legs lock straight. Stay relaxed.

● Move down into a comfortable squat, bending your knees. Allow your movement to come from your hara.

● As you reach the ground and come into a full squat position, the swaying becomes very slight.

● In the full squat position, connect to the receiver as ki comes down the legs. Breathe out and totally relax. This is a point of stillness.

relax ▶ ▶ ▶ **relax** ■

leg meridian stretches

These positions work the leg in different stretches to open the meridian flow. Doing this encourages the movement of ki.

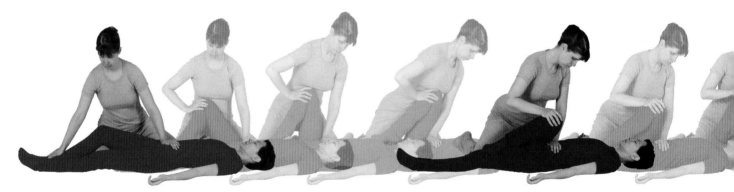

● Start with the spleen stretch by opening the receiver's leg out to the side, with her knee hooked over your leg for support. The toe on the foot of the receiver's bent leg should touch the ankle of their opposite foot.

● In an open base cezar position, place your mother hand on the hara and the child hand just above the ankle on the side of the shin bone. Keep your hara central to the middle of the stretch.

● Hook your hand under the bent knee and slide the leg up and back. Breathe and hold for a moment. Your body provides strong physical support for the leg being stretched. Listen to the receiver to see how comfortable the stretch is.

● Bring the knee across the body, over the hara as far as is comfortable. Lean over the receiver, keeping your hara over the area you are working on. This stretches the side of the thigh, the gallbaldder meridian.

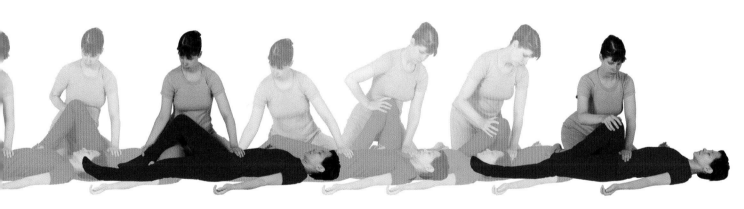

● Ease the leg back to the starting position, with the knee hooked over your leg, but bring the heel of the receiver's bent leg to their opposite knee. Drop your hand to the ankle. This stretches the small intestine meridian.

● Allow the receiver's leg to straighten slightly by letting it slide down your leg. Place your hand on her knee and press it up toward her chest, coming up onto your own knees as you do so.

● Bring the receiver into a gentle side stretch by moving her knee across her body.

● Now go back to "rocking in hara and down legs" on pages 56–57 and repeat on the other leg.

▶   ▶   ▶   **repeat**   ■

palm up chest from hara

Palming up from the hara connects the hara to the heart energy. This technique grounds the emotions and is very calming. It can also be reversed, bringing energy down to the hara for a deeper calming effect. However, avoid using this technique if the receiver is distressed or upset, as they may find it too invasive.

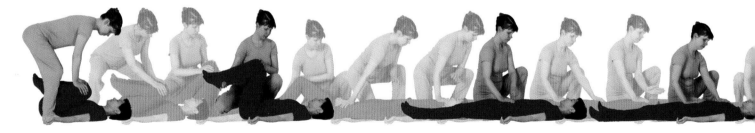

● Start with the receiver's knees pressed to the chest. Your own knees should be bent and your back relaxed.

● Move to a position alongside the receiver, half-turned toward her body, in a semi-squat. Bring the receiver's legs down, supporting them with your right leg, which should slide out to the side as you do so. Your hara should face the movement.

● Lower the receiver's legs down to the floor completely. You should be side-on to the receiver, one knee up, one down. Place one hand over the mid-line of the hara. This is a point of stillness, so pause and tune in to the receiver's body.

● Put your other hand (the child hand) above the first, on the mid-line. Palm up the chest. As you reach the breast area, use the side of your hand instead of the palm. Listen to the receiver's body as you work. Pause if it is kyo; move on if it is jitsu.

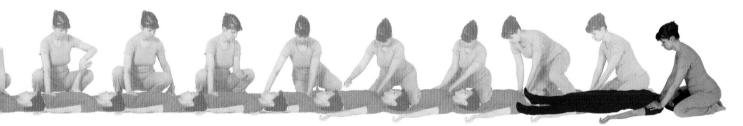

● When you have worked up to the top of the chest, move your child hand to hold the receiver's palm. Try to feel ki between your two hands. This is a point of stillness.

● Keeping in contact with the hara, move the receiver's arm out to the side and come into a squat position. Start to palm the top of the shoulder.

● Start to move around to the top of the receiver's head. Place both your hands on the top part of the chest, just below the collar bone.

● In the cezar position, with your legs either side of the receiver's head, place your hands on the top of the shoulders and press down to release tension. Breathe out as you do so.

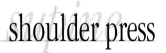

shoulder press

The shoulder press is good for relieving tension in the shoulder area. It also opens

up the lungs, relieves neck tension, and stops the back from hunching.

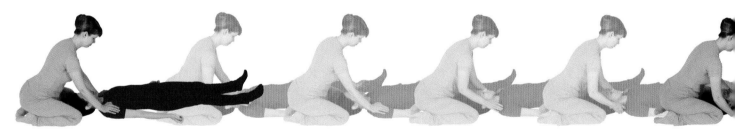

● Start in the cezar position with your hands on the receiver's shoulders, as shown at the end of the previous page.

● Pad down the tops of the shoulders with the heel of the hand, as for catwalk I (see pages 30–31).

● Stay relaxed as you work. Padding in this way opens up the upper body for deeper work.

● Shuffle back slightly. Slip your hands under the receiver's neck and cradle the base of the skull so your fingers curl up into the neck. Allow the weight of the head to fall into your hands rather than trying to grip it.

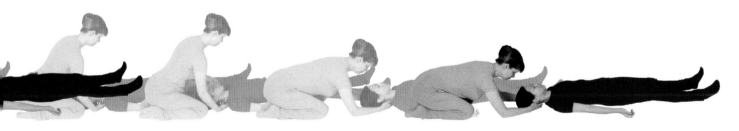

● Using your fingers, work down either side of the vertebral column toward the shoulders. Support the head with your energy; work with the intention of giving the head support.

● Continue to work down the neck. Be aware that the head and neck are connected to the body, so your work will have an impact beyond the area you are touching. You are not just working on a disconnected head.

● Come back up the neck and work along the ridge at the base of the skull, where it joins the neck. Gently press your fingers into the natural indentations at the base of the skull.

● Come to a point of stillness while cradling the head. Allow your fingers to rest on the base of the skull.

arm stretches

Arm stretches open up the meridians in the arm. These meridians are the heart, bladder, lung, spleen, heart protector, liver, and kidney. These stretches also encourage the flow of ki.

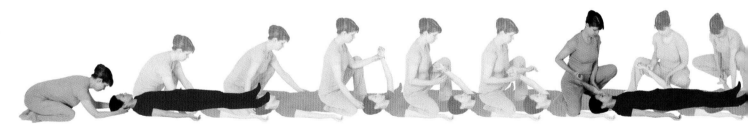

● Start by cradling the receiver's head, with your fingers touching the base of the skull, as described on the previous page.

● Shuffle forward and come up onto one knee. Reach for the receiver's wrist and keep ki contact by placing your other hand on the top of her head.

● Holding an upright position, bring the receiver's hand around toward you in a circular motion like the movement of the hands of a clock. Shake the arm gently to relieve any tension.

● Support the receiver's arm by placing it on your leg. Bend the arm at the elbow. Move one hand down the arm to below the elbow and allow its weight to drop into your hand, rather than gripping it. Keep your other hand on the wrist.

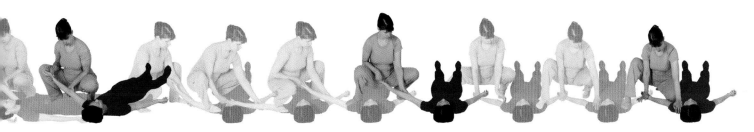

⬤ Bring the arm back toward its original starting point as if moving around a clock face. Move with it and support it in a squat position as you do so.

⬤ Continue to work around the clock face, moving with the arm. Reverse the knee positions as you move in the squat position.

⬤ Start to move as close to the receiver's body as is comfortable. As you come to the receiver's side, move the supporting hand from the elbow to the dip just below where the collar bone joins the shoulder.

⬤ Place the receiver's arm on the floor with one hand on her shoulder and the other on the edge of her thumb. Keeping firm pressure in both hands, feel a connection between your two hands. This is the lung stretch.

▶ ▶ ▶ **breathe** ▶

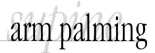

supine arm palming

Palming down the arms is a good way of working on the meridians and feeling for kyo and jitsu.

As you work, practice feeling for the connection between your two hands.

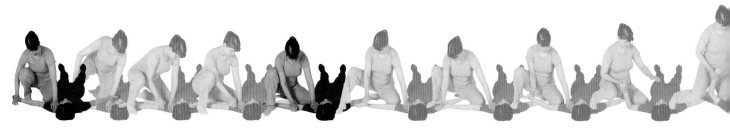

⬤ Start off in lung stretch position, with one of your hands on the receiver's shoulder and the other on the edge of their thumb, feeling a connection between your two hands.

⬤ Move the receiver's arm at a right angle to her body. With one knee raised to form a wide base, keep one hand on the shoulder and place the other next to it. Start to palm down the center of the arm. This is on the heart protector meridian.

⬤ Palm down the arm at a slow pace, feeling for kyo and jitsu. The heart is an emotional center so be aware of the receiver's reactions as you work.

⬤ Palm all the way down to the end of the middle finger. Use your own fingers to work on the receiver's finger—your hand will be too large for such a small area.

▶   **ground**   ▶   **breathe**   ▶   ▶

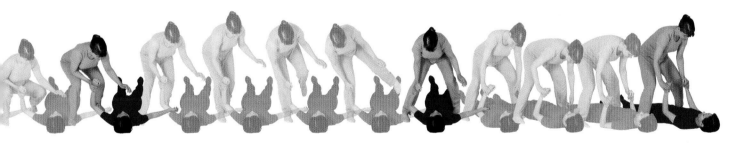

● Hold the receiver's hand loosely by the wrist and raise the arm, coming up into a kneeling position. Move your mother hand from the shoulder, but stay in contact energetically.

● Come up into a semi-upright position and step over the receiver. Remain grounded, with your legs quite wide apart.

● Reach down for the other arm, keeping your knees bent, and hold this arm loosely by the wrist as well.

● Hold both the receiver's arms loosely by the wrists. Stay relaxed as you do so. This is a point of stillness.

stay connected   ▶   ▶   ▶   **relax**   ▶

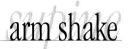

arm shake

The arm shake loosens the shoulder girdle and is good for increasing mobility around the neck and shoulder area—a part of the body that often suffers from tension.

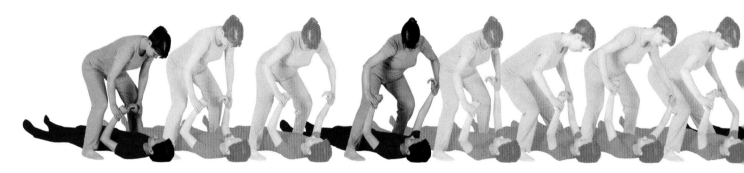

● As described on the previous page, hold the receiver's arms by the wrists and remember to keep your own hands relaxed. You should be grounded, with your knees slightly bent and your back relaxed.

● Stay loose and generate a figure-of-eight movement from your hips and your hara. Move the receiver's hands in the same pattern, backward and forward. Bend your knees as you shift your weight from side to side.

● It is very important to keep loose and relaxed—this is more important than the size of the movement.

● Continue to work in the figure-of-eight in an easy, relaxed way.

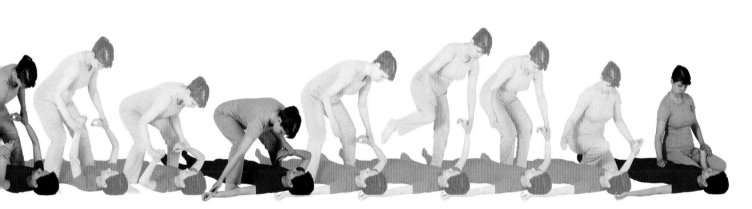

● Gradually, make the movement smaller and smaller as you lower the receiver's arms. Bend over as you come down and remember to keep your knees soft as you do so.

● Bring the movement to a halt completely and put one of the receiver's arms down gently.

● Step over to the side of the receiver's body, still holding one arm and keeping in energetic contact with the other.

● Kneel into the cezar position, close to the receiver, with one hand on the receiver's hara and the other on the palm, which should be resting on your leg. This is a serene, supportive position. Go back to "shoulder press" on pages 72–73 and repeat on the other arm.

▶ **stay in contact** ▶ ▶ **breathe** ■

side turn

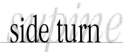

This technique turns the receiver over onto her side, so you can work in the side position. This is a very good position for working on people with stiff joints and big muscle structures. It is also good for working on pregnant women in their second and third trimesters; however, avoid working on women who are in their first trimester of pregnancy.

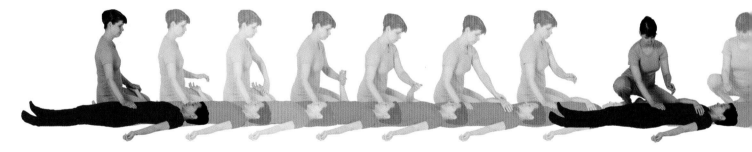

● As on the previous page, start off in the supportive contact position. Place one hand on the receiver's hara and the other on the palm, which should rest on your leg.

● Tell the receiver you are going to move her. Lift the arm on your leg by the wrist.

● Place this hand on or just under the receiver's chest. Keep your other hand on the receiver's hara.

● Bring your other hand down to the hara and swap hands. Turn your own body (from your hara) to face the point at which you are working on the receiver. Hook your free hand under the receiver's knee.

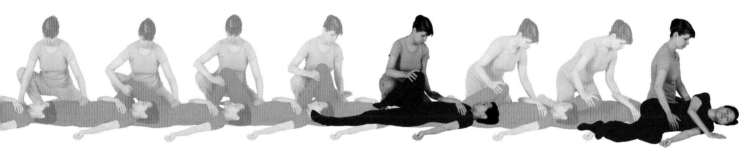

● Bring the receiver's leg up, bending at the knee. Use your raised knee as a support for the receiver's leg.

● Let gravity pull the receiver's knee over her own body and roll the receiver's body with it. Place the hand on the hara just under the shoulder to give a little push.

● Guide the movement all the way over until the receiver is on her side. Support her head with a pillow.

● Put your hand back on the receiver's hara and place the other hand in the middle of the back, in between the shoulder blades on the spine. This is the heart diagnostic area. Feel for a heart–hara connection between your hands.

▶   ▶   ▶   connect   ■

side

shoulder loosening

This technique is good for loosening the shoulders, the shoulder joint in particular. It also relieves stiffness in the neck that arises as a result of tight shoulders.

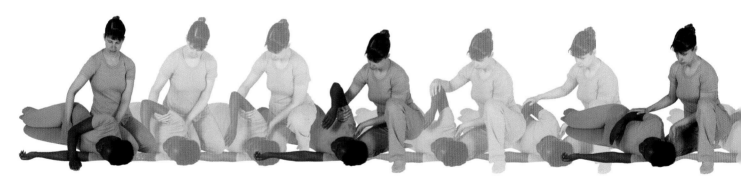

● In the cezar position, place your mother hand on the receiver's hara and the child hand on the edge of her shoulder blade.

● Bring your mother hand up and slip it under the receiver's arm, lifting and supporting her upper arm with the inside of your forearm. Your other hand comes onto the top of the shoulder.

● In a semi-squat, pull the receiver's arm back and slide your fingertips under the edge of the shoulder blade. Keep your upright knee against your elbow to support and push your arm and fingertips into the shoulder blade.

● Move your supporting arm up toward the receiver's elbow, raising the receiver's arm, and work along the whole of the edge of the scapula. Move from your hara not your shoulders.

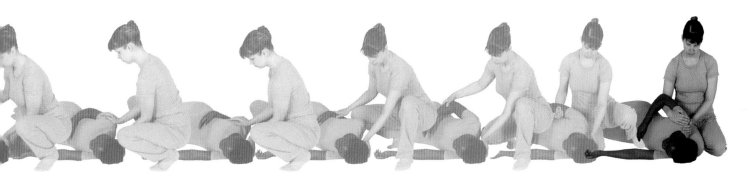

● From a squat position, let the receiver's arm down and move so your hara is facing the top of the shoulder. Place one hand on the end of the shoulder, the other where the neck joins the shoulder.

● Catwalk with the heel of the hands, one hand, then the other, on these two points. Push the shoulder down toward the receiver's waist.

● Bring one hand down to the receiver's elbow and the other to the top of the shoulder.

● Slide your arm under the receiver's arm to join the hand already on the shoulder. Gently interlock your fingers to hold the receiver's shoulders. Listen to the receiver's shoulder joint.

shoulder rotations

Shoulder rotations open up the shoulder blades and stretch and loosen all the muscles around the shoulders—an area that can often be very tense.

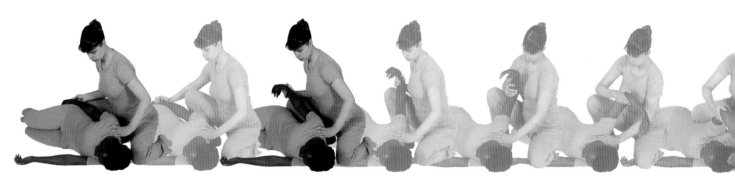

● Start with your raised knee behind the receiver's body and your bended knee down behind the head. Place your raised leg against the receiver's buttocks or lower back to provide support. Place one hand on the receiver's shoulder.

● Bring your knee out from behind the receiver and place your other hand on the receiver's arm.

● Straighten up slightly and start to lift the receiver's arm, holding it under the wrist.

● Moving from your hara, start to rotate your own body. This will rotate the arm you are holding. Work within the receiver's range of movement. The hand on the shoulder is there to listen to the receiver's body. Here, a very flexible receiver is shown.

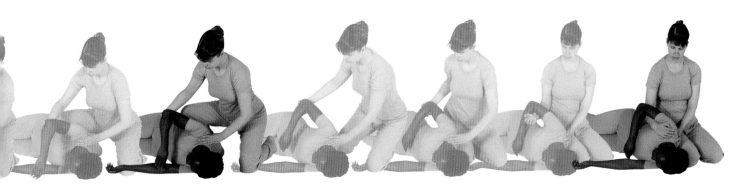

● Be secure in your own base. Adjust your position as necessary so you can work comfortably as the receiver's arm rotates. As the rotations become larger, move your hand from the wrist to the elbow. This provides better support for the receiver's arm.

● Reduce the size of the rotations, keeping your arms and shoulders loose and relaxed. Stay focused and breathe into your hara.

● Prepare to release the arm and place it on the side of the receiver's body. Turn your hand under the elbow to guide it down and come into the cezar position.

● Allow the hand under the receiver's elbow to move up toward the shoulder and join with the hand already there. In this hugging position, listen for any changes around the receiver's scapula and shoulder area.

▶ **breathe**　　　▶ **listen**　　　▶　　　　■

palm down arm

The outside of the arms tend to be jitsu, particularly on the gallbladder meridian, so palming can be stronger and faster than on the inside of the arm. However, listen to the receiver to make sure that this generalization is true for them.

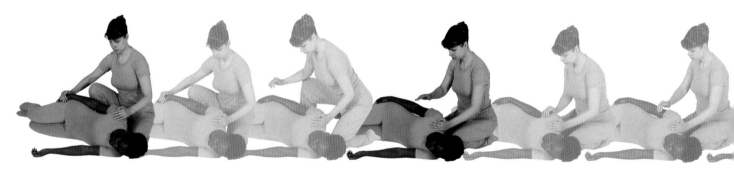

● Place one hand on the top of the receiver's shoulder. With the receiver's arm on their side, place your other hand on their hand. With one knee raised and one knee down, support the receiver with the raised knee and stay earthed.

● Come up into a more upright position and move back slightly so you can comfortably work on the receiver's arm.

● Move your hand from the receiver's hand to the top of her arm. Stay in energetic contact as you do so and move into the cezar position.

● Start to palm down the middle of the outside of the arm.

earth ▶ **connect** ▶

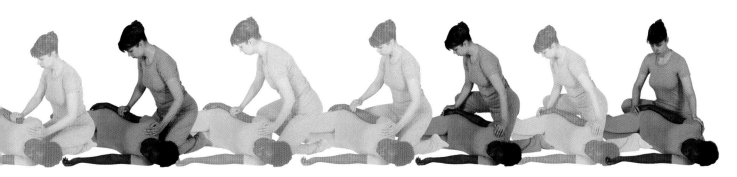

● Listen for the quality of ki in the receiver's arm. Palm harder for tight muscles where there is lots of jitsu. You may need to use a slight amount of extra body weight to do this. Check with the receiver that this does not become uncomfortable.

● Work all the way down the arms and hands to the fingers at the end of the meridian.

● Palm down the top of the middle finger. Raise one knee to support yourself as you cover the distance from hand to hand. Use your fingers to work on the receiver's fingers—your hands will be too large.

● Your hands should finish back in the starting position, with one on the shoulder and one on the receiver's hand, lined up along the meridian.

listen ▶ ▶ ▶ ▶

side upright arm extension

The side position is excellent for stretches that are not possible in other positions. This technique is a very effective stretch down the side of the body on the gallbladder meridian.

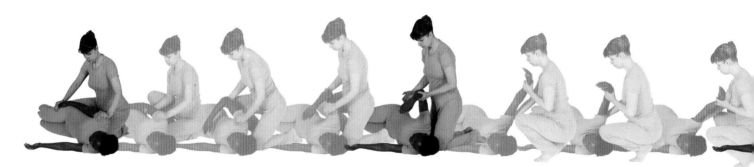

● Start off with one knee raised and the other down. Place one hand on the receiver's shoulder and the other on the receiver's hand. Listen to the receiver.

● Hook your hand under the receiver's elbow and start to lift the arm. You will need to move back slightly to allow the receiver more space in which to stretch.

● Come up to kneel on one knee and bring the receiver's arm up toward her head. This should be a gentle movement. Move your hand on the shoulder to the hook of the elbow. The hand currently on the elbow will move to the wrist.

● Move to a position behind the receiver's head and at a slight angle, coming down into a squat as the receiver's arm comes down. Place one hand on the shoulder joint (the mother hand) and use the other to hold the wrist.

▶   **connect**   ▶   ▶   ▶

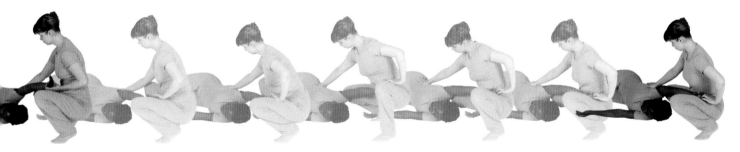

● Fully extend the receiver's arm, keeping the elbow slightly bent. Let the receiver's hand rest on your knee for support. Keep your other hand (the mother hand) on the shoulder.

● Take your mother hand down the side of the receiver's body to facilitate a full stretch.

● Coming up into a semi-squat, place the receiver's arm on the top of your thigh. Try to feel an energetic as well as physical connection with the receiver's arm through your thigh. Be careful not to overstretch the receiver.

● Bring your hand up to the side of the armpit, keeping the receiver's outstretched arm supported by your thigh. Drop down into a deep squat.

listen ▶ **connect** ▶ **breathe** ▶

side upright arm stretch

This technique stretches the gallbladder meridian down the side of the body. When the arm is taken to an upright position, it stretches the heart protector meridian.

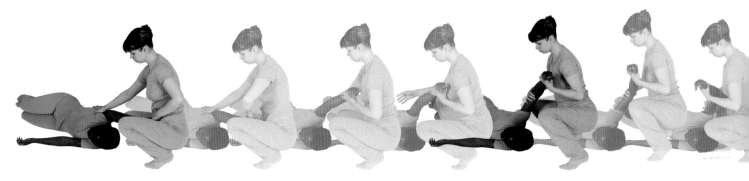

● As on the previous page, bring your hand up to the side of the armpit, keeping the receiver's outstretched arm supported by your thigh. Drop down into a deep squat.

● Start to lift the receiver's arm away from your hara and move one hand to just under the elbow. Hold this arm loosely by the wrist with the other.

● Allow the receiver's arm to relax so it bends slightly.

● Start to move behind the receiver, still in a squat.

▶ **relax** ▶ ▶ **breathe** ▶

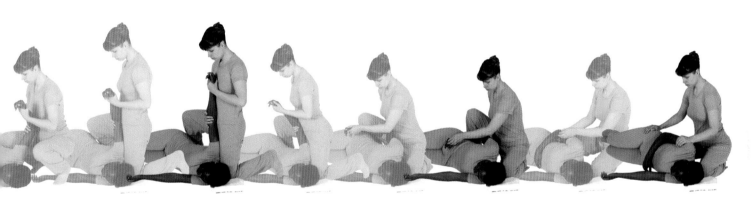

● Move fully behind the receiver. The receiver's arm should be at 90 degrees to her body, with the arm slightly bent.

● In a semi-squat, fully straighten the receiver's arm, supporting it with your body. This contact allows you to listen to the receiver's body and lets you know if she is comfortable. Then, gently extend the arm upward.

● Start to lower the receiver's arm, bending her elbow, and come down into a lower squat as you do so. Place the arm along the side of her body.

● This is a point of stillness, with one hand on the shoulder and the other on the hip. Sit in a wide-based cezar position.

▶ **extend** ▶ ▶ ▶

forearms opening torso

This technique opens up the muscles down the side to the body. It also opens the gallbladder, triple-heater, and large intestine meridians.

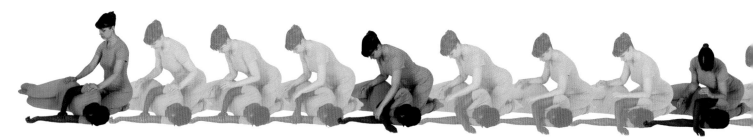

- Position yourself behind the receiver, in the cezar position. Place one hand on the receiver's shoulder, the other on the hip. Breathe, ground, and relax.

- Move back slightly and bring your chest forward. Move one hand off the shoulder and use your forearm instead of your hand on your hip.

- Reach down for the receiver's arm to move it up and out of the way. This will give you room to work on the side of the receiver's body.

- Press down on the side of the receiver's body with your forearms. Push and pull your forearms gently backward and forward to create the massage movement. Work up and down the side, moving one arm, then the other.

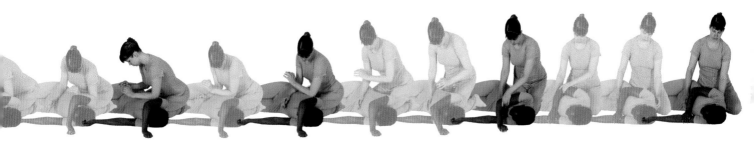

● With one forearm on the hip and the other on the area under the armpit, push your arms apart to create a stretch along the length of the receiver's side. This also prepares the area for work with the elbows.

● Use the point of the elbow for work in areas that feel tight. However, the side is a sensitive area and elbow work may be too strong, so ask for the receiver's feedback. Use the forearm of the other arm to provide support by placing it on the hip.

● Move the arm on the receiver's hip down so your hand rests on her hara. Also, move the receiver's outstretched arm to a more relaxed posture under the chest.

● Keeping your hand on the receiver's hara, move the other to the space between her shoulder blades and feel for the heart—hara connection between your two hands.

back palming

This gentle side-position technique is less dynamic than other techniques. It is good for deep listening work.

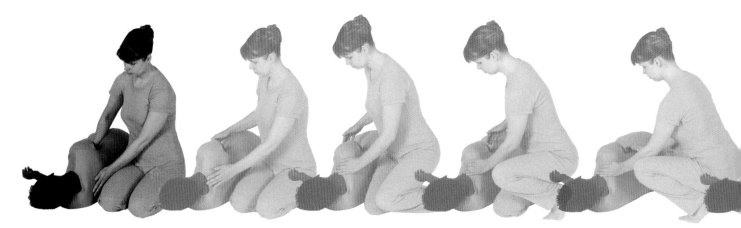

● Start in the position demonstrated on the previous page, with your hands on the heart–hara connection. Stay earthed in the cezar position with your leg in contact with the receiver's back. This is a very calming and supportive position.

● Prepare to move face-on to the receiver's back. Move the hand on the hara to the kidney area of the back. Keep this hand in energetic contact with the receiver as you move it. Bring your other hand to the receiver's shoulder for support.

● Move into a squatting position face-on to the receiver's back.

● Listen to the receiver with your hands.

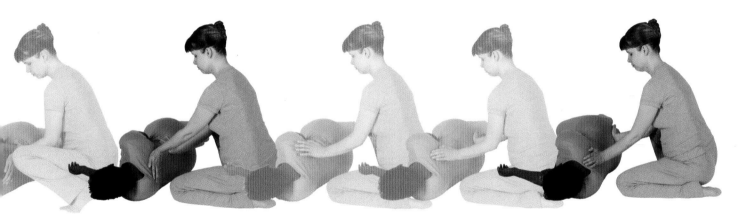

 Drop down into a semi-squat with one knee up and one down. Put your hand on the back in between the shoulder blades, on the heart area. Listen for kyo and jitsu.

 Start to palm down the top edge of the spine, 1.5 cun from the middle of the spine, listening all the time as you work.

 Hold your hand for longer on areas where you find kyo and palm to disperse areas of jitsu. As you work, move your other hand to the receiver's sacrum.

 When you have finished working down the spine, move the palming hand back up to the top of the spine, with the other hand still on the sacrum. This is a place of stillness, so ground and listen.

connect ▶ ▶ ▶ **ground** ▶

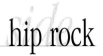

side hip rock

The hip rock encourages the flow of energy around the sacrum and sexual organs and is associated with sexual energy. It also loosens stiff hips.

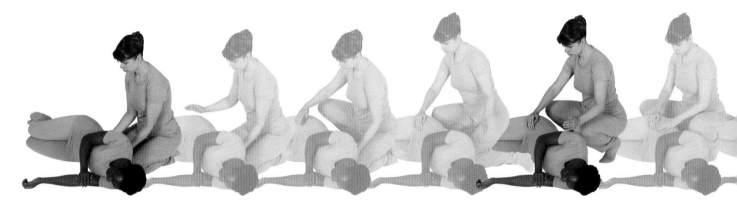

● Start in the same position shown on the previous page with one hand on the top of the spine and the other on the sacrum. Kneel down into the cezar position.

● Move the hand on the receiver's sacrum to the hip bone. Keep in energetic contact as you move.

● Come up into a more upright position, squatting on your toes. Stay earthed and grounded and breathe deeply.

● Shift your weight from your toes to the soles of your feet—you need a solid base to work from to move the receiver. Stay centered in your hara and keep one hand on the receiver's hip for support and balance.

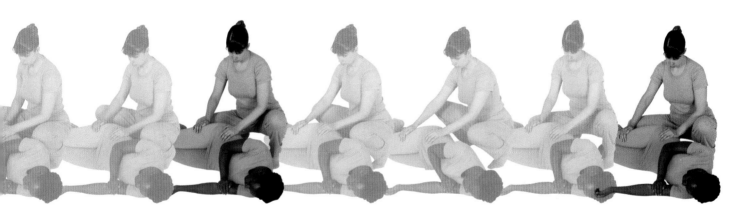

● Move both hands to the receiver's hip and rock it backward and forward. Start to move one hand down the receiver's leg to develop the rocking into a larger movement, where appropriate.

● Listen to the receiver's movement with your hands and follow their movement.

● If the receiver's movement starts to feel more free and loose, move your hand down the outside of the thigh to further expand the rocking motion.

● Slowly decrease the movement until you come to a stop, reaching a point of relaxation.

side leg rotation

Leg rotations open up the joints of the hip. This is a very useful technique for encouraging extra mobility and is also used to relieve symptoms associated with arthritis and rheumatism.

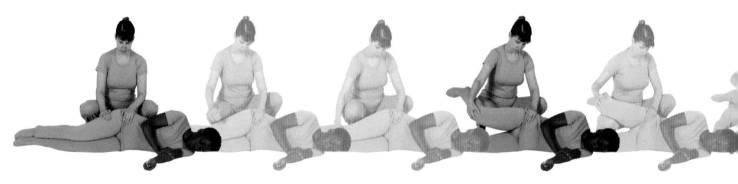

● Start in the position demonstrated on the previous page, squatting behind the receiver with your hands on the hip and outside of the thigh.

● Hook your hand under the receiver's knee and start to lift the leg. Make sure you are close to the receiver so you do not overstretch.

● As you raise the leg, quickly slip your leg under hers for support. This means that your leg, rather than your arm, takes the weight. Keep your hand on her hip as you do so, listening in to the receiver.

● Start small rotations of the leg, pivoting from the receiver's hip, going in the easiest direction first. Guide the leg with your own leg, not with your hands. Your hara should be facing and leading the movement.

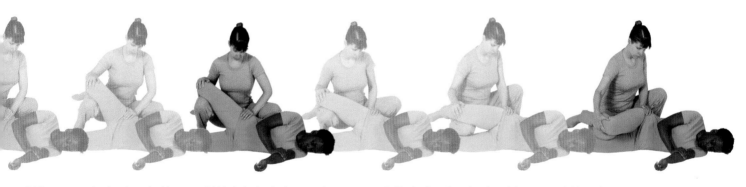

• Use your mother hand on the hip to check whether more rotations are needed. It may be possible to open up the hip more.

• Work the leg in the opposite direction, starting with small rotations.

• Gradually reduce the size of the rotations before coming to a stop, using your leg to carry as much weight as possible. Only use your arm at the last moment to guide the receiver's leg back down.

• Listen in to the receiver and check for changes in ki in the leg.

▶   ▶   ▶ **relax**   ▶

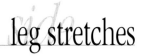

leg stretches

The leg stretches shown here are very useful for opening up the
muscle groups and meridians on the outside of the thighs.

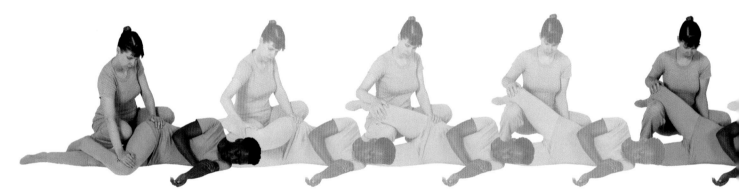

● In a low squat position, place one
hand on the receiver's hip and the
other just above the knee, pressing the
receiver's upper leg down and across
the other. This stretches the center of
the outside of the thigh and the gall
bladder meridian.

● Hook your hand under the
receiver's knee and start to bring the
leg up. As in the previous technique,
quickly use your own leg to support
the receiver's leg.

● Continue to raise the leg, elevating
your knee to lift and support it. This
stretches the front of the thigh and
the earth meridians.

● Continue the stretch by gently
pulling the receiver's leg back toward
you. Move your hand to the receiver's
sacrum to listen and support—this is a
strong stretch.

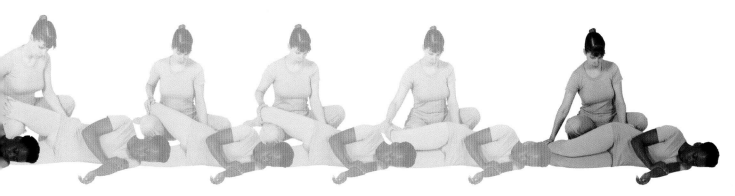

Start to bring the receiver's leg back down by lowering your knee. As you work, you will stretch the triple-heater meridians.

As the leg comes down further, you will reach the stretching points for the stomach and spleen meridians. Remember to take the weight of the receiver's leg on your knee.

Guide the receiver's leg down until it is resting on top of the other.

Place one hand on the lower leg just above the ankle and your other on the outer edge of the buttock. This tunes in to the gallbladder meridian and is a point of stillness.

▶   ▶   ▶   **relax**   ■

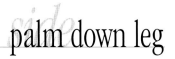palm down leg

This technique works the gallbladder meridian, which can be jitsu. You can use the elbow as well as palming techniques in a faster, deeper way here, but check with the receiver that this feels comfortable.

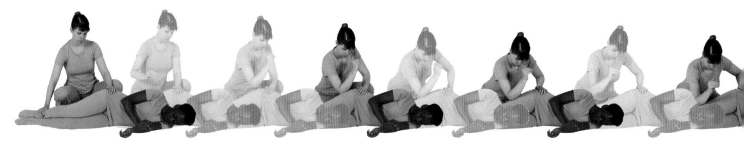

⚫ In a squat position, place your mother hand on the receiver's hip and the child hand on the side of ankle just above the foot. Tune in and listen.

⚫ Turn slightly so your hara faces the area to be worked. Use the point of your elbow and ensure your mother hand is strongly connected to the elbow.

⚫ From a wide, firm base, start to work your elbow down the middle of the outside of the thigh. Remember to work from your hara, not your shoulder.

⚫ As you work down the leg, lower the base you are working from so you are not compromised into working from your shoulders.

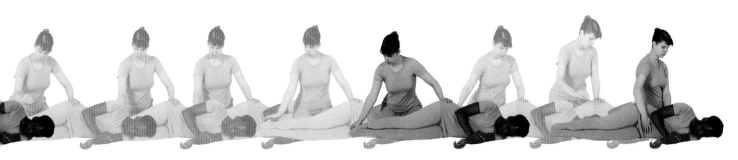

● Finish your elbow work on the knee, keeping your mother hand on the hip. Come into an upright position, facing the receiver's leg.

● Start to palm down the outside of the lower leg, from the knee downward, tuning into the receiver's ki.

● Finish working down the leg, coming to stop with one hand on the hip and the other just above the ankle. Listen in to the meridian and notice any changes.

● Come side on to the receiver so your hip bone is touching their sacrum. Place one hand on the kidney area and the other on the hara. Connect your two hands. Turn the receiver onto her other side and repeat, starting at "shoulder loosening" on pages 84–85.

▶   ▶   ▶   **connect**   ■

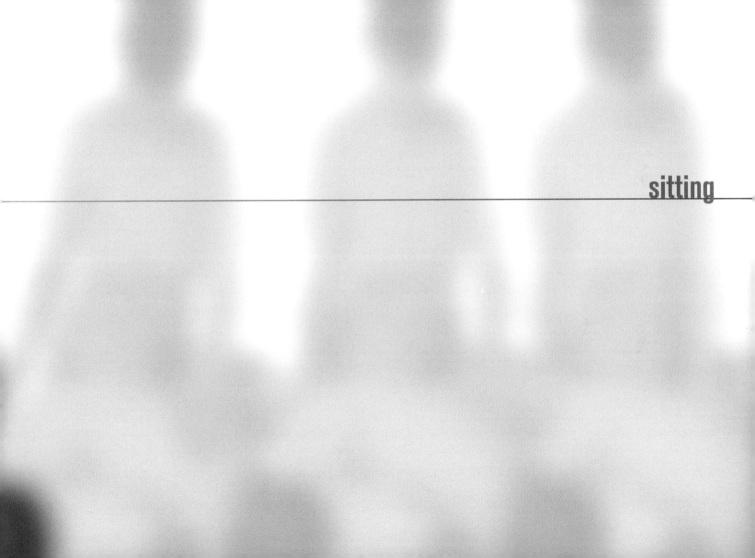

sitting

kneeling, connect shoulders, palm down back

This technique opens up the receiver's back and is good for feeling kyo and jitsu.

It is also good for preparing the back for deeper work.

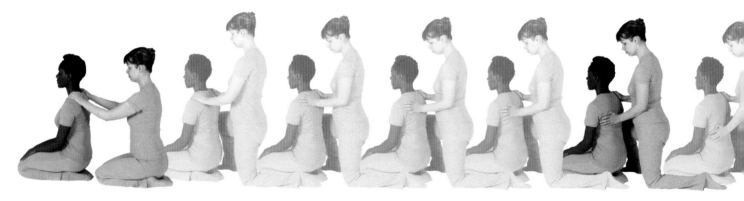

● Start in the cezar position, behind the receiver, with both hands on the receiver's shoulders.

● Come into an upright position, with one knee raised and one knee down, listening with your hands.

● Positioned at a slight angle to the receiver for room to work, start to palm down the receiver's back, 3 cun from the center of the spine. Work with your fingers turned out, listening to the different qualities of ki.

● If you feel kyo, think about the corresponding area in your own body. Visualize the area opening up and try to extend that ki back to the receiver.

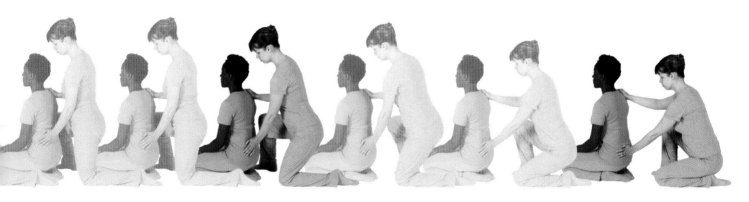

● Expand and experiment with this technique, and listen carefully to the effects in the receiver.

● Continue to work in this way to the end of the receiver's back.

● Finish with one hand on the sacrum and the other on the receiver's shoulder. Listen.

● Reverse your knee position and start to work on the other side of the spine, from the top down. Remain in ki contact with the receiver as you change hands.

▶ **visualize** ▶ ▶ **listen** ▶

elbow points down shoulders

This technique relaxes the shoulders and is very useful for alleviating the tension often generated by sitting for long periods in an office. It is good for encouraging energy to drop back down into the body from the shoulders. Make sure you use the points of the elbow when working.

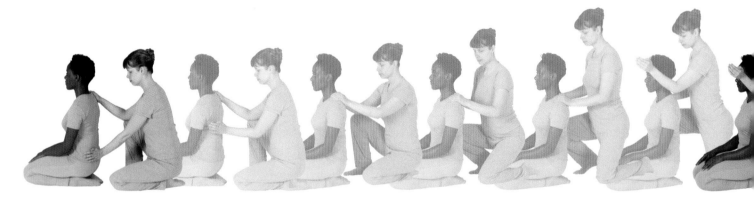

● Connect to the receiver before starting and make sure you are earthed and breathe deeply. Place one hand on the receiver's kidney and the other on their shoulder, resting your elbow on your knee. Listen.

● Bring the hand that is on the kidney up to the receiver's shoulder, staying in ki contact as you move the hand. Get as close to the receiver as is comfortable—if you sit too far away you will overstretch.

● Start to come into an upright position, with one knee raised and one knee down. Keep listening.

● Prepare to use your elbows on the tops of the shoulders. Work on one shoulder at a time, staying in—and working from—your hara.

▶   **connect**   ▶   **listen**   ▶   **earth**   ▶

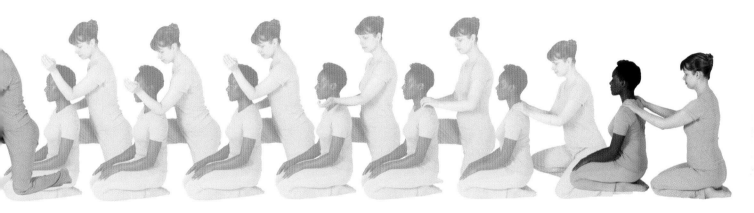

● Using the point of the elbows, work along the band of muscle on the top of the shoulder.

● Continue to use the point of your elbow, working outward to the edge of the shoulders.

● Reverse your knee position and repeat the elbow work along the receiver's other shoulder.

● Bring your hand back to the shoulder and sit back deep into your hara. The more relaxed you are, the more relaxed the receiver will be.

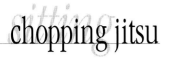

sitting
chopping jitsu

This technique is very effective for dispersing jitsu. It is a dynamic, invigorating movement that breaks up muscle tension and energy held on the top of the back.

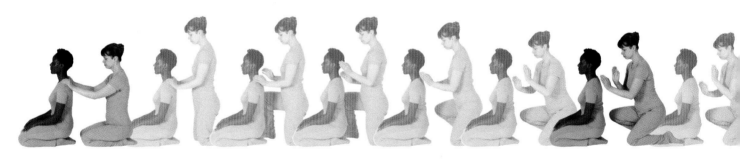

● Start in the position illustrated on the previous page, kneeling in the cezar position with your hands on the receiver's shoulders.

● Come up onto your knees; then raise one leg so that the knee is bent.

● The chopping technique involves working with the edge of your hands. Keep your wrists loose so you do not simply hit the receiver and make sure that your shoulders are relaxed.

● Work along the tops of one of the shoulders and the area in between the shoulder blades.

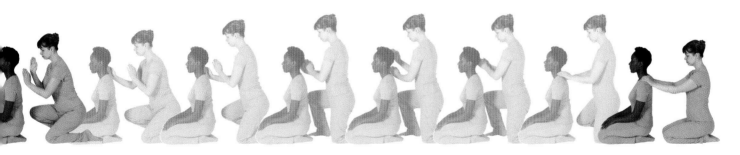

As you work down to the area between the shoulder blades, start to sit back, bending your knees and keeping your back straight.

Work on the reciever's other shoulder. Make sure that the chopping action does not become mechanical—stay grounded and breathe deeply.

Slowly decrease the chopping motion and gradually bring it to a stop. Place both your hands on the receiver's shoulders.

Return to the cezar position; connect, breathe, and earth.

▶ **breathe** ▶ ▶ **relax** ▶

sitting arm rotations

Rotating the arms opens up the shoulder joint. It also relieves tension in the shoulder area and promotes flexibility and range of motion.

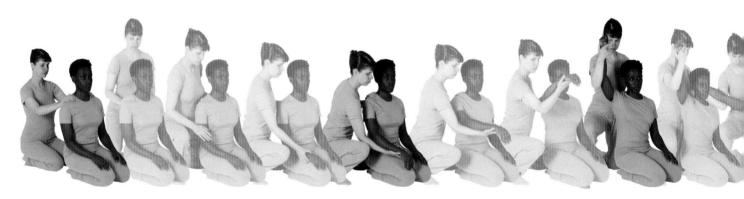

● Start in the position illustrated on the previous page, kneeling in the cezar position with both hands on the receiver's shoulders.

● Come up onto your knees at an angle of 45 degrees to the receiver's back. Place your left arm on the back of the receiver's right shoulder and move your other hand onto the receiver's right arm.

● Sit back into a squat and slip your hand under the receiver's right hand. Allow its weight to fall into your hand rather than just gripping the wrist. Give the arm a short shake to release any tension.

● Supporting the receiver's arm, lift and move it back, raising it above the head. Come into an upright position behind the receiver on one knee. Listen with the hand on the shoulder to learn how far to raise the arm.

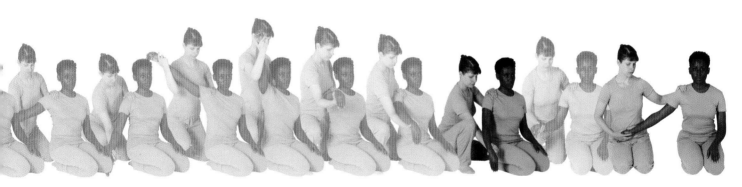

● Start to rotate the arm backward, moving your own body with the rotation. Remember to move from your hara. Come down to a lower squat as the receiver's arm lowers.

● Rotate the arm the other way, listening to the receiver to make sure you are not overstretching the arm.

● Bring the arm back down to a point of stillness.

● Move to a position parallel to the receiver, holding her arm out with her hand on your hara and your supporting hand still on her shoulder. Repeat on the other arm.

guitar thumbing down arm

Using your thumbs to work down the arm is another useful way to open up the meridians in the arm. When working, practice connection, intention, and feeling for kyo and jitsu.

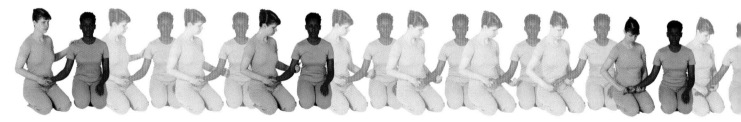

● Start in the same position as illustrated on the previous page, with the receiver's hand on your hara and one hand on the receiver's shoulder, listening.

● Wrap your hand around the receiver's arm as if you were holding a guitar. Start to work down the center of the arm, on the heart protector meridian. Keep the receiver's other hand on your hara and listen.

● Either use all your fingertips or just one, using the others as support. Work all the way down to the end of the middle finger, pausing on areas where you feel kyo.

● Raise one knee to support the receiver's arm and prepare to work down the outside of the arm.

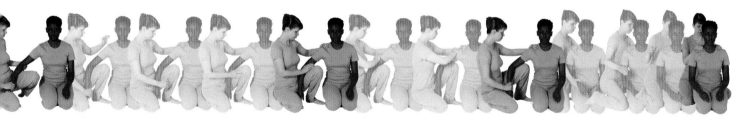

● Let the receiver's arm drape over your supporting leg. Place one hand on the wrist and the other on the shoulder. Start to work down the center of the outside of the arm.

● Work with either your fingers or palms. The outside of the arm is generally jitsu, so you can work harder and faster, but check that this is comfortable with the receiver. Work down to the end of the middle finger, along the gall bladder meridian.

● Moving from your hara, come around to a position behind the receiver and gently place her hand back in her lap. Repeat the whole technique on the other arm.

● When you have finished working on both arms, come back behind the receiver with your hands on her shoulders. Feel for any change in the receiver's energy. Breathe and relax. Repeat on the other arm.

▶   **relax**   ▶   ▶   ■

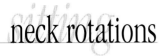

neck rotations

Rotating the neck is very effective for loosening stiff muscles and helps to relieve tension in the head. This slow and unwinding action is good for preventing headaches, but the technique should not be used if the receiver actually has a headache.

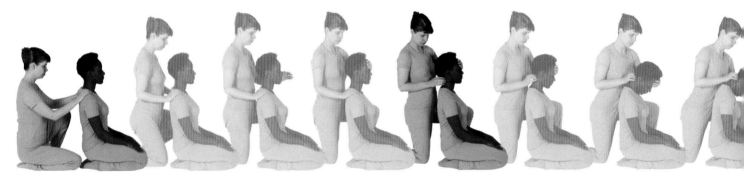

● Start off in the same position as illustrated on the previous page. Place both hands on the receiver's shoulders and semikneel.

● Get closer to the receiver to support them energetically and raise yourself onto one knee. Bring one hand around to the receiver's forehead, so her neck does not have to work. Stay grounded.

● Your hand should hold the head gently, but supportively. Move your other hand to the top of the receiver's neck, putting your thumb and first finger on the two indentations at the base of the skull—located either side of the top vertebra.

● Allow the receiver's head to drop forward slightly. Follow the movements of the receiver's head, rather than being the guide, and listen. This should be a very slight, slow movement.

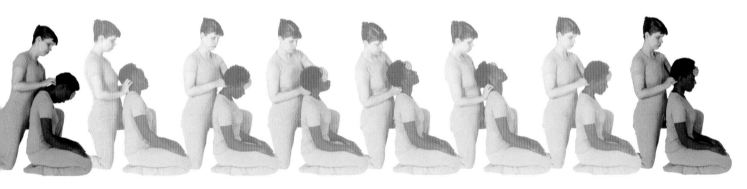

● Keep following the receiver's natural movement and continue to listen.

● The receiver's head will lead you one way and then the other, in no particular order or direction. The movement can be become larger and more open as the receiver wants.

● The movements of the receiver's head will gradually become smaller. Follow them to a natural stop.

● Once you have come to a stop, feel the connection between both your hands and listen for ki passing between them.

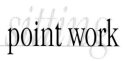

point work

Point work is very useful for working the bladder meridian in the neck. It is also used to disperse tension in the neck and is especially useful for those who work in an office at a computer or who spend long periods watching television.

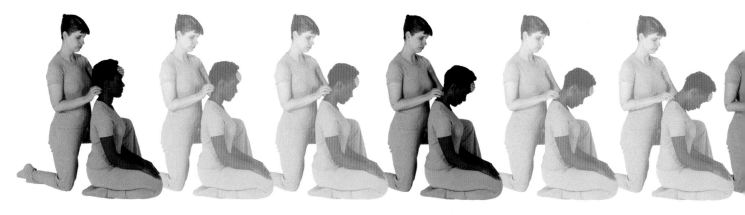

● Start in the position illustrated on the previous page, with one hand on the receiver's head and the thumb and forefinger of your other in the two indentations at the base of the skull.

● The starting position at the base of the skull is called bladder 10 and is a clearing point. Working on this point brings clarity to the mind, relieves headaches and nasal congestion, and promotes concentration.

● Start to work down the neck, 1.5 cun from the center of the spine, using the thumb and first finger.

● Listen as you work and feel the receiver's body respond.

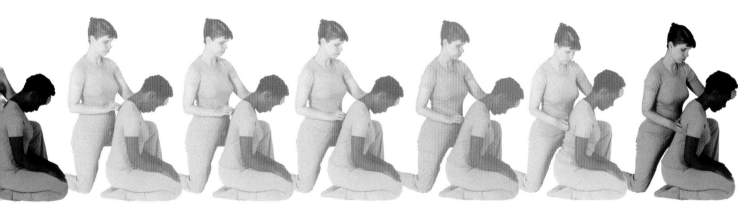

● Work down the neck as far as the top of the first vertebra in the back. You can feel this protruding slightly as the receiver's head is tilted forward. Remain grounded and breathe into your hara.

● When you have reached the top vertebra in her back, start to take the receiver into an assisted cat stretch.

● The cat stretch stretches the back and is relaxing and regenerating.

● Ask the receiver to lean forward. Support her with your hand on the head as she starts to come down. You will have to move forward with her.

listen ▶ breathe ▶ stretch ▶ ▶

cat open stretch

This stretch is a traditional restorative yoga pose using supportive shiatsu techniques to facilitate deeper opening in the back.

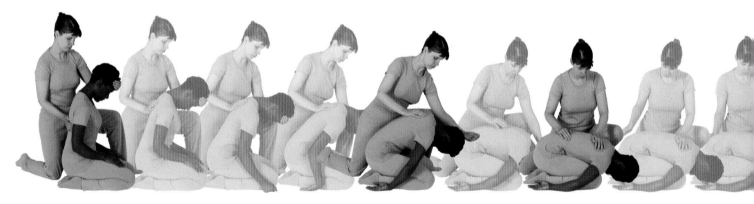

- Allow the receiver to come forward completely until her chest is resting on her knees, which should be apart. You can support her head with a firm pillow if this is not comfortable for her.

- Move into a low, semi-squat beside the receiver. Place one hand just under the scapula on one side of the spine and the other just above the sacrum on the opposite side.

- Start to move your hands around the back, pushing them in opposite directions. Start by opening up the lower back and kidney area. Move on to disperse tension in the upper back.

- Keep in your hara and stay in a solid, open-squat position so you are comfortable when working.

▶ relax ▶ ▶ breathe ▶

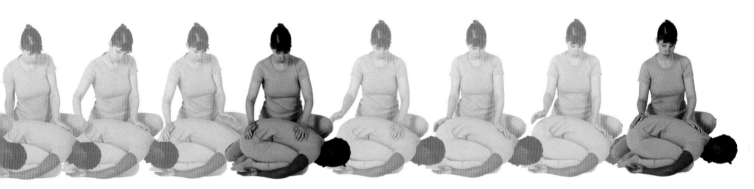

● Remember that this is a relaxing technique. Keep this in your intention when working.

● Continue to work around the receiver's back, opening up the whole area.

● Gradually reduce the size of the stretches in preparation for palming.

● Listen to the receiver's body and encourage ki to flow through the kyo areas.

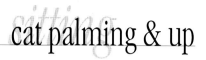

sitting cat palming & up

The intention of this palming brings ki to the kidney and sacrum area. This is a very calming technique and moves ki away from the adrenal glands and into the kidneys.

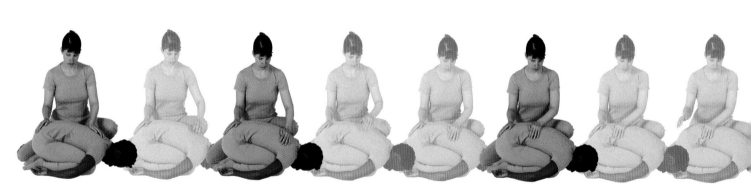

● From a semi-squat position with the receiver bent forward, place one hand on the kidney area and the other on the sacrum. Try to make contact with the receiver's ki. Breathe into your hara and listen.

● Visualize ki filling the kidneys and sacrum. Move your hands around the lower back as appropriate to the different sensations you feel.

● As you work around the lower back, pay particular attention to the area around both kidneys.

● When the receiver's body feels completely relaxed and you feel she has taken what she needs, prepare to bring her upright but ask first if she is ready.

breathe

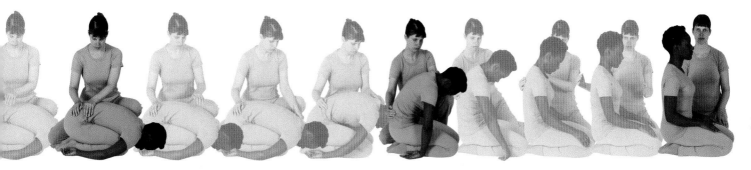

● Place one hand on top of the receiver's shoulder and the other on the kidney area to support the receiver as she rises.

● When the receiver is almost upright, move one hand to her forehead and the other to the heart area in between the shoulder blades. Come into a more upright position as the receiver comes up.

● The receiver should stay relaxed as she comes up. Focus your intention to facilitate this.

● Slowly take your hands off the receiver, supporting her with your ki, before coming into your own space and allowing her to be in hers. Finish in the cezar position.

▶ **listen** ▶ ▶ **relax** ◼

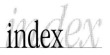

index

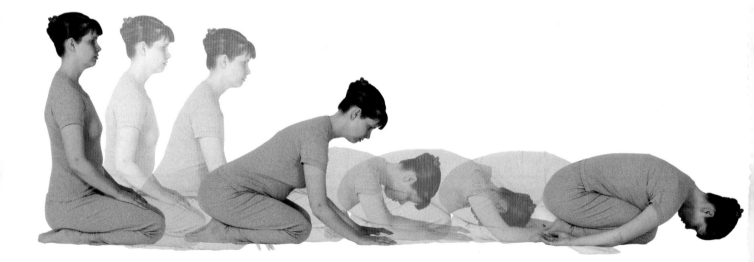